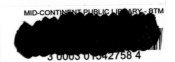

By Tosca Reno

The Butt Book

The Pan-G Non-Surgical Face Lift: Bodybuilding for Your Face

The Eat-Clean Diet

The Eat-Clean Diet Cookbook

The Eat-Clean Diet Workout

The Eat-Clean Diet Workout Journal

The Eat-Clean Diet for Family & Kids

The Eat-Clean Diet for Men

Tosca Reno's Eat Clean Cookbook

The Eat-Clean Diet Companion

The Eat-Clean Diet Recharged!

The Eat-Clean Diet Stripped

The Eat-Clean Diet Cookbook 2

Just the Rules: Tosca's Guide to Eating Right

The Eat-Clean Diet Vegetarian Cookbook

The Start Here Diet

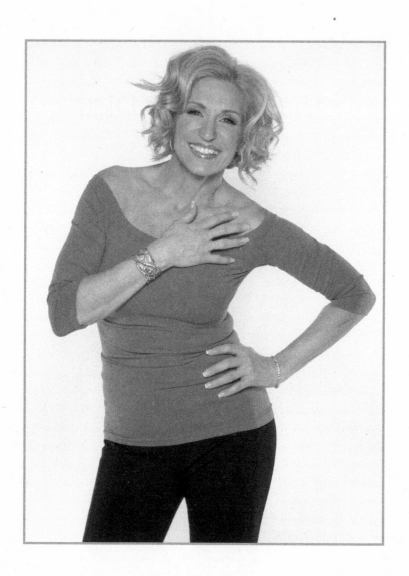

The Start Here Diet

*Three Simple Steps That Helped Me
Transition from Fat to Slim . . . for Life*

TOSCA RENO

with Billie Fitzpatrick

Ballantine Books | New York

This book proposes a program of diet and exercise recommendations for the
reader to follow. However, you should consult a qualified medical professional
(and, if you are pregnant, your ob/gyn) before starting this or any other fitness
program. Please seek your doctor's advice before making any decisions that
affect your health or extreme changes in your diet, particularly if you suffer
from any medical condition or have any symptom that may require treatment.
As with any diet or exercise program, if at any time you experience
any discomfort, stop immediately and consult your physician.

Copyright © 2013 by Tosca Reno

Published in the United States by Ballantine Books,
an imprint of Random House,
a division of Random House LLC,
a Penguin Random House Company, New York.

BALLANTINE and the HOUSE colophon are registered
trademarks of Random House LLC.

LIBRARY OF CONGRESS CATALOGING-IN-PUBLICATION DATA
Reno, Tosca.
The start here diet : three simple steps that helped me transition
from fat to slim . . . for life / Tosca Reno with Billie Fitzpatrick.
pages   cm
Includes index.
ISBN 978-0-345-54801-6 (hardcover : alk. paper) —
ISBN 978-0-345-54802-3 (ebook)
1. Reducing diets—Recipes. 2. Weight loss. I. Fitzpatrick, Billie. II. Title.
RM222.2.R463 2013
641.5'635—dc23   2013020752

Printed in the United States of America on acid-free paper

www.ballantinebooks.com

2 4 6 8 9 7 5 3 1

First Edition

Book design by Virginia Norey

I dedicate this book to you, one of many who are searching for their best selves. You are not alone. The time is right to fly. I have been there too and am in flight with joy over my new life and the possibility for you to have it, too.

Contents

Introduction

I'm Tosca Reno, the mom of four who went from fat and frumpy to slender, healthy, and sexy—all *after* age forty. You may know me as the author of the *Eat-Clean Diet* franchise, the *New York Times* bestselling author of *Your Best Body Now,* or the creator of the diet lauded by celebrities such as Angelina Jolie, Nicole Kidman, and Halle Berry for helping them shed their post-baby weight. You may recognize me from *Good Morning America, CBS Sunday Morning, Access Hollywood,* or one of the hundreds of other media and personal appearances I make as I travel around the United States and Canada inspiring people to lose weight, get fit, and become healthier.

If you're reading this book, then you probably already know a little bit about me. But with all the time that I've spent on the road, I am just beginning to find out about *you.*

I always assumed that the people who bought my books were those who mirror the person I am *today*—totally committed to a healthful lifestyle and the changes necessary to achieve it. But what I'm learning is that the majority of my books are purchased by people who are more like who I was when I *began* my journey.

I didn't always look the way I do now. For years, I was a fragile pawn in my own yo-yo dieting nightmare, in which I spent the majority of my life starving myself, bingeing, and trying every diet known to mankind to lose weight and fit into my pre-kid jeans, all to no avail. I was seventy-five pounds heavier than I am now, then I got a little thinner, then got fat again. Up and down went the scale. I stayed in this limbo for more than twenty years before finally figuring out that I had the power to not only lose weight but keep it off and get healthy.

But like most stories that seem to fit into neat nutshells, the version that I have told up until now only touched the surface of my experience. Indeed, the life I have described in my other books is a somewhat sanitized version of what really happened to me; what I've shared before only hints at the real struggle I went through and that millions of people—perhaps including you—still endure. And for reasons that will soon become clear, it is only now that I have the courage and power to dig deep and be fully honest about what had to change inside of me before I could truly transform my life. I hope that sharing my experience and my journey to a healthy weight will inspire you to travel the same road—the road to happiness with the way you look and feel— because to be truly successful in reshaping yourself is to find the why first. Why are you not at your ideal weight? That answer is paramount.

It's not that I have some shocking, tabloid tell-all to reveal. My story is epically relatable. Nearly 130 million people in the United States alone live just like I did: terrified of making changes, without the know-how to stop their self-sabotaging behaviors.

I am not only a former fat girl, a woman who stayed up late to avoid being caught eating ice cream and peanut butter and hunks of cheese. I am also a woman who was tangled up in a bad relationship and so many folds of fat that I no longer knew who I was. I had lost a sense of where I ended and others began. Sound familiar? I was a member of what I fondly call the "invisible millions." I couldn't see myself clearly; I felt lost and humiliated; I was hiding from myself.

Most stories that have at their heart the loss of our true selves have one of two endings: we either find ourselves or we continue to muddle through our lives—sad, powerless, and often very, very overweight and very, very sick.

I found myself. But not without wrestling with what was at the center of my fear of change. At first, I had no power to stop eating certain foods that were sabotaging my life and my health. I was so fearful of adjusting even the slightest thing in my day that instead I stayed immobile—stuck physically, emotionally, and spiritually. Then slowly I gained clarity and courage. I began to feel less threatened by small changes. I began to listen to another voice within me.

If you, too, belong to the "invisible millions," if you, too, can't seem to move off the couch—literally and metaphorically—I hope that my full story and the Start Here process for change will finally inspire in you the confidence and courage to change your life forever. I hope it is the spark for your personal renovation. If I can do it—you can do it.

The Start Here Diet is a simple three-step process. It's gentle and easy and brought me out of my dark, lonely, and heavy place, the place where you must begin, too.

Part 1, "Coming Out of Hiding," turns your focus inward. Many diets begin by asking you to identify your goals, such as the number of pounds you want to lose. My strategy is a bit different: I want you to focus on what's *behind* your weight gain and *behind* your desire to lose weight. No diet will ever be successful if you don't go to that place inside you, a place usually wrapped in pain, discomfort, shame, self-defeating habits, and fear. Unless you take care of this inner place, this inner fat person who is hiding from the world and herself or himself, then no matter what the diet, it will not work in the long run.

And I am all about the long run. I am all about showing you how you can—and will—heal that inner place, that part of you where your gifts and secret strengths reside.

As a former overweight person, I know what the prison of extra pounds does to the heart and the soul, never mind the body. And I know that for you to emancipate yourself from the prison of too much weight, to get in touch with the real you and the gifts that lie within you, you must face the intense fear and discomfort that surround you and that are presently dictating your life though you may be unaware of this vise-grip.

Step 1 will help you do this. I call this step your *dive inward*. I will describe my own dive inward and then ask you to get in touch with *your* heart, ask yourself some tough questions, and find some ways to forgive yourself, give yourself permission to move on, and begin to dismantle the pain that keeps you in your prison.

This first, heart-focused step is not complicated, but some of the questions you will ask yourself, and the changes they lead you to, probably won't be easy. However, they are absolutely necessary and build a foundation from which you can take the subsequent two steps. Diving inward is the foundation for the beginning of your permanent weight loss. It is the step that will put you on the path to losing the ten, twenty, fifty, one hundred, or two hundred pounds that have you locked up, unwell, and miserable. Diving inward is where I started my process.

Part 2, "Losing Weight and Regaining Yourself," lays out the details of the next two simple steps—sometimes I even call them "baby steps." *Removing your hidden food* (step 2) and *moving a little* (step 3) are rooted in gentleness and simplicity. I know neither of these steps asks you to do anything you can't do.

Identifying your hidden foods is much simpler than it may sound. We all have foods in our kitchens that too often find their way to our plates. We know they are less healthy than they could be, and if you're honest with yourself, you know that these foods (or just one ingredient) are the ones you reach to for comfort. For me it was peanut butter (which isn't inherently "bad" unless, like me, you are eating it late at night and straight out of the jar with a spoon) and ice cream. I reached for these foods when I was alone—I reached for them to give me pleasure, the pleasure and confidence I was missing in the rest of my day. Your hidden food(s) weigh you down physically and emotionally; clearly seeing the frequency with which they turn up in your diet and beginning to replace them with healthier options is a simple yet amazingly effective baby step toward huge weight loss. I will also introduce you to my kitchen shortcuts, which will help you rethink the way you shop, allow you to put together a meal or snack, and offer tools so that you are ready to deal with obstacles, troubleshoot roadblocks, and reach for and find support where and when you need it. The kitchen, too, is a good place to start your own process.

Don't be intimidated by "moving a little" either! I appreciate that you are busy with your work or with your home or with your kids or with all three. I appreciate that most people don't have any "extra" time they can devote to exercise. But I do know that you can add small movements to your housework or when sitting at your desk, and those small extra movements *are* exercise. In this step, I ask only that you add small movements to what you are already doing. I offer fifty movements that count as exercise, fifty movements from which you can find a handful that will become part of your daily routine. Moving more is a painless and ultimately joyful way to start your weight loss journey.

Part 3, "Renovating Day by Day," offers you twenty-eight days of meals as well as twenty-eight days of activities that require as little as fifteen minutes a day. The eating and activity plans are meant to be flexible, so that you can either follow them as a literal guide or use them as inspiration to create your own food and exercise combinations.

Part 3 also includes an entire chapter that helps you develop support tools so that no obstacle will sabotage your plans and goals. The book ends with thirty easy and absolutely delicious recipes that you can make at home. They apply to you, the busy woman who is probably not a chef, just like me!

A big part of succeeding at this diet is keeping close track of your physical and emotional progress, and to do that I'm going to ask you to practice journaling.

The inner part of your journey needs a safe place in which to unfold. So it's really important that you keep a journal—a place where you can put down your feelings, fears, words of encouragement; a record of all you experience as you begin this process of uncovering your gifts and your secret strengths. This is the beginning of you telling your own story.

And because I think this piece is so integral to your process and your success, I am going to share with you selections from my own journal. I think it will be valuable for you to see that I was a lot like you not so long ago. I hope you find encouragement, support, and solace in that knowledge. Not only will you see how uncomfortable I felt, but you will also see how, day by day, and with small steps, the changes I wished for myself became real.

Your journal is not simply a log where you record the foods you eat every day, though that is part of it. The journal is the place where you ask yourself questions about why you are hiding, begin to look at the inner part of you where your gifts reside, and start to understand your relationship with food. This journal becomes your story.

This journal can be a spiral-bound notebook with lined pages, a Google doc on your computer, a Notes page on your smartphone, or even a blank book in which you draw as well as write. You can even keep an audio journal by using a video or tape recorder to house your story. Your journal can take many shapes or forms; what's most important is that you create it and use it.

Your journey through this diet might get intense at times. Yes, it's simple; I've made the steps as uncomplicated as possible. But I know that taking these steps and making the changes can be hard! Even thinking about making changes can cause anxiety and make your heart race. Keeping a journal is one way to help manage this experience. Keep it close, by your bed or near your favorite chair. Think of your journal as a place to empty your worries and rediscover the real you, the one who's been in hiding. It's the place where you can reconnect with a part of yourself that may have been buried for a long time.

Throughout the chapters that lie ahead, from time to time I will remind you to turn to your journal. Having that safe, private place to dive into your heart and bare your soul is wonderfully liberating. I still keep a journal today! Remember, if you don't write it down your desires never become reality.

This is a book for all of you who feel so profoundly stuck on the couch that you can no longer even imagine moving your body. This is a book for all of you who feel trapped by your bodies and who refuse to look in the mirror. Perhaps you've lost the sense of your body's shape and size. Maybe you have always struggled with your weight, or maybe it was the act of quitting smoking or the birth of your children that left you with extra pounds you haven't been able to lose. Regardless of the trigger or original cause, I believe that diving inward, discovering your hidden foods, and moving just a little is the right plan to kick-start you into a new way of life and into caring for yourself and your body again.

So come join me. I will show you how to trust yourself again, forgive yourself, and imagine changes you thought were beyond your reach. You will see how I and others like me began by taking baby steps to change our lives. And then you will be more ready than ever before to take the three gentle, easy baby steps that will lead you to permanent weight loss and tremendous health. Let the journey begin!

PART ONE

Coming Out of Hiding

1

My Prison

Many of us think we are being honest when we say to ourselves, "I'm happy." We think we are being honest when we tell ourselves and those we love, "I'm fine" or "Don't worry, everything is all right."

But often we are lying. Not on purpose. Not because we want to mislead others. But because we are in such pain, or feel so uncomfortable with how we look or how we feel, that we hide. We hide from our families, our friends, our doctors, our co-workers. We hide from ourselves. We hide because we feel ashamed. We tell everyone that we feel fine because how could we possibly admit that we are not?

For years, I lived my life in hiding, and coming out of hiding took some painful reckoning. When others asked how I was doing, I would reply in a defensive tone, "I'm fine!" The message I clearly sent with that response was "Don't dig any deeper. Leave me alone."

When I was seventy-five pounds overweight, I was heavy emotionally as well as physically. I gained the weight because I was out of touch with my inner needs and voice; remaining heavy was a way to continue hiding. Admitting and recognizing the power of that inner place is where my journey to permanent weight loss and health began. And it will be the same for you. Not the same story, but the same reaching inward to the place where you've been hiding.

To understand my weight loss journey you need to also understand what *else* I had to lose—small step by small step—before I could shed pounds and find *my true self.*

I grew up in Kingston, Ontario, Canada, with three siblings, one sister and two brothers. We had a happy home and my parents were loving and supportive. My dad was resourceful, reliable, and sturdy. But it was my mom who was in charge of things. She was strict and she set high standards for me and my siblings; she wanted the best for us all and pushed us to achieve.

I was always a strong-willed young girl. I loved the challenge of competition. I was an athlete—I ran, swam, and played soccer. I loved horses. I was always on the move, rarely looking behind me as I forged ahead into my next new adventure. Always in a rush, I sometimes didn't look ahead either. I had more than a few run-ins with telephone wires and bushes and tree roots!

At university I studied science. I also fell in love hard and fast when I was just twenty years old. Since my then-love was a couple of years ahead of me academically, I interrupted my studies when he graduated and together we went out west. I believed in his dreams for our success and for our future together. We were married when I was twenty-three—not unusually young for the time, but definitely an age when I was only just beginning to understand myself.

I didn't question giving up further education for my husband's career: it seemed natural, something I could do to show him the depth of my love and commitment. Besides, didn't I have the rest of my life to figure out what *I* wanted to do?

But very early into my marriage, my connection to myself began to disappear. I cannot tell you about one specific moment, or even one particular event that triggered my separation from myself. It was a slow build. But day by day, month by month, I began to lose a sense of my own importance. It probably began with the very simple act of giv-

ing up what had been important to me—studying science—for someone else's dream.

Even as I was thrilled to have children, I think I really let go of the
real Tosca when I became a mother. Like many women (of all ages), I
jumped into parenthood and all its responsibilities and quickly became absorbed in making other people happy. What I can see now is
that when I focused so completely on caring for my kids, I stopped
knowing how to care for myself. But that wasn't the only reason I
began hiding.

Early in my marriage, we moved a lot for my husband's job. The
moves were necessary for his career, but they were also disruptive and
I was more or less solely responsible for the logistics of each move and
for helping the kids adjust each time. I loved my husband; the heavy
lifting was a way of showing my support. But each move was stressful
and each one took a lot out of me. It should have been goodwill that
was building in our partnership, but instead there was mounting ten-
sion, and I felt I had to walk on eggshells. A lot of the time, especially
at home, I felt nervous and vulnerable. This emotional environment
made me withdraw from myself even more. It didn't feel safe to simply
be me. Even now as I describe it to you, the reader, I realize I was then
and am still afraid to admit that my relationship was transitioning
from love to routine, and ultimately to something very different from
love; it was abuse.

When I was twenty-seven, I gave birth to our second beautiful
daughter. Soon thereafter, we moved yet again, the seventh time in ten
years. Again, I felt enormous joy bringing forth this new life into the
world. But I was beginning to realize that there was a darkness creep-
ing in and around me. I was busy, busy, busy and yet never made time
for myself. My movements kept me out of my head and out of my
heart. I scurried around for others. I wanted to think everything was
perfect. I began to tell myself, "Everything is fine." "You should be

grateful." But somewhere deep inside me I knew these words were just not true. And on the surface life was indeed grand. I loved our house, our great community, our pretty little suburban neighborhood. I got wonderfully lost in being a mom. I loved being with my girls and teaching them about school, life, and themselves. Isn't this what I needed to make my life meaningful, my heart feel safe and purposeful?

The surface never tells the whole story. In reality, with each passing day, month, and year, I was becoming less happy, less relaxed, more stressed, and more sad. I found myself relying on destructive ways of covering my anxiety and dulling my own yearnings. "Time for myself" was time spent eating. I had a warped sense of what it meant to indulge my own needs!

My bad habits consumed me. Some of these habits may even seem familiar to you. I stayed up late after everyone went to bed, made myself comfortable on the living room sofa, and lost myself in a quart of ice cream or a jar of peanut butter. Swallowing one spoonful after another, I no longer tasted the food or felt the pleasure of its sweetness. Rather, I shoveled in food to obliterate my own feelings of sadness. My husband and I had drifted far apart—he busy with work and I busy managing the house and family to a self-imposed perfection. I berated myself if the house was messy or if there were things left undone at the end of a busy day. These late-night feed-fests were a way of battling back the feeling that I was a loser. I was desperate to block out the constant, gnawing fear that something was terribly wrong with me, with my life. One of the most basic human needs, according to Tony Robbins, master life coach, is the need to feel significant. Caring for everyone else was meaningful work and had my marriage been happy, I might have felt differently, but all I knew then is that the care and feeding of other souls didn't satisfy my own soul's need for significance.

When I got married, I weighed about 127 pounds—thin for a woman of my height (5'8"). But ten years later, the number on the scale had reached two hundred and four pounds. I was a bloated and obscured version of my former self.

At two hundred plus pounds, I avoided mirrors and cameras. I hid myself in big, bulky clothes. Everything about my body made me feel awkward, ill at ease, not good enough. The photo on this book is one of the only ones I have of myself at that time—it's not that I threw them all away, but rather that I rarely stepped out from behind the camera to allow myself to be photographed! I didn't want to document my unhappy weight. I didn't want to document my sad truth.

In addition to simply gaining weight, I also started to be physically unwell. On several occasions I even passed out. This was hypoglycemia at work—my organs were beginning to complain about my poor diet. My blood sugar would soar, then plummet, taking its toll on my entire body. I was often sweaty, clammy, and dizzy. I sometimes had heart palpitations—an irregular heartbeat that caused a tightness in my chest. This really scared me because my father had suffered from heart disease all his life, and ultimately the disease took him from this world. I didn't want the same fate for me and my kids.

As perhaps you know, food has a terrible way of being both a problem and a solution. With each passing day, month, and year, I continued to use food to calm me but also to squelch my dreams and block out my thoughts of my future. The more I ate, the more I felt further diminished, unworthy, and dependent. I had trouble even remembering who I had been as a girl and young woman before I married. Some days, I would quickly glance at photos from my childhood. The images staring back at me of the smiling, strong, confident girl had nothing to do with who I had become. Yet most troubling of all was that I couldn't figure out how to connect the dots: I knew I ate too much, but how, really, had I become this person staring back at me in the mirror?

Not surprisingly, I was on edge all the time, and I took even a passing comment about my weight as a deep criticism about me as a person. I saw disapproval in other's eyes. And I heard a nasty voice in my ear: "You look fat today." "Why are you wearing that blouse?" "Those jeans don't exactly flatter you." "Are you crazy or something?"

How had I become this sad, overweight, powerless woman? And what was I doing to myself? Where was my belief in my own power?

The bigger I got on the outside, the more I retreated into my litany of self-criticism. I resisted listening to a deep part of me who wanted that frank inner conversation—about my marriage, about my future, about what *I* wanted to do with the rest of my time on Earth. I was depressed, lonely, and powerless to seek help. In truth I didn't know where to look. I needed this book all those years ago but there wasn't anything like it at the time of my crisis.

This feeling of paralysis kept me stuck in my destructive, repetitive behaviors. I didn't realize these negative patterns were part of the prison I was building around myself. There were rare occasions when I allowed myself to peek out and have fun, usually with my children, but most of the time I was introverted and quiet.

I focused on the girls, wanting only to keep them safe and happy, and their busy lives provided good cover. But was this real? Was this even good for the girls if it was so wrong, so bad, for me?

Of course, children always see more than you want them to—they knew I was unhappy. They knew something was not right in the house. Because I was not taking care of myself, because I was eating fatty, sugary foods that sapped my energy, I was compounding an already bad situation.

I am certain many of you can relate to that experience: our families are our priority, but it's a slippery slope from taking care of others to neglecting ourselves. It becomes—without our even realizing it—somehow more comfortable to put the needs of others before our own. And to be sure, this "giving up" and giving so much of ourselves feels good—it's one way we can show our love for others. But of course there are many ways to show our love for others that don't compromise our own needs and hopes and dreams. I didn't realize that then at all. In a way, I think that I shifted into sacrifice mode so that I could mask my own fears of being who I was. But sacrifice comes at a price, and mine was to become emotionally, physically, and spiritually depleted.

Today of course, I know that true beauty and happiness do not come from the outer appearance so much as from what is radiating from deep inside. But at this time in my life, I had not yet discovered this clear truth. It's curious to me how what you put out in the universe is what you receive. When I was younger, in my twenties and thirties, I was nothing but an envelope of negativity, and that is exactly what I got back. It did not occur to me to operate from love and gratitude. I didn't know where to look for positive support or a reality check; I didn't even realize that I needed a reality check because I was completely convinced that I knew where I stood and that I was a bad person for getting to that place. I was convinced that I was worth nothing. The more I internalized this thinking, the worse I allowed others to treat me. It was a vicious cycle. I stayed bound in this kind of thinking for years, actually allowing others to treat me badly, further tightening the chains around my spirit. Soon, though, I was going to take a profoundly simple step: I was going to look inside myself and gather my courage to believe that I did matter. I was about to dive inward.

But in those early days, the only voice I heard was small and squeaky, telling me not to take up so much space. *Hide,* the little voice told me. I suppose if I were really in a prison I would curl up in a ball in the farthest corner and keep myself from view. The dominant feeling I was experiencing was shame. I was ashamed at myself for being a failure, fat, insignificant, and worthless. This was not the way I was raised or the person I had expected to be. I had allowed myself and others to destroy my purpose.

Deep down, I knew something was wrong with my life. If I had had the courage to be honest with myself at the time, I would have admitted that what was wrong was my marriage: it had soured beyond repair. My husband and I had drifted worlds apart and weren't supportive or communicative with each other. I was not happy and I did not feel respected, truly loved, or cared for. I felt uneasy in my own home, too vulnerable to relax and be myself. But even as I am now sure that my husband was as much to blame as me, I still thought I was the one in the wrong. I doubted my own instincts: *Are things really that bad? Maybe I am just holding myself to impossible standards. Don't all women feel this way about marriage after a while?*

I would try to justify my feelings, my fear of change, always arriving at the same conclusion: *You don't have what it takes to live a different kind of life. You owe it to your family to try harder and stay with them.*

So I soldiered on, and kept on eating in a silent battle with myself.

Food was the only personal joy I had. Food had become my medicine, my best friend, my only safe, reliable source of comfort. After all my work for the day was done, after everyone else was in bed, I retreated to the living room sofa. I might turn on the television; sometimes I read magazines and dreamed about faraway places that looked exotic or romantic. But then I closed the cover and settled in to eat my quart of ice cream, hunk of cheese, or spoonfuls of peanut butter again and again—and, often, all of them together.

Sometimes I was scared I would be caught eating, and I actually hid in the closet for fear that my husband would angrily criticize my eating and my weight. He had a temper and I was often the target for it. He thought my overeating was a deep flaw and a sign of weakness, and I believed he was right about me. I felt ugly, unsexy, and worthless. He didn't contradict me or help me think otherwise. My late-night trysts with food had become one of the few sources of pleasure in a life that was becoming increasingly unsafe. Under cover of darkness, I thought no one would notice what was becoming of me.

It's not like I didn't try to get out of this mess of an existence. I didn't try to leave the marriage—which would have been the healthy and self-loving thing to do—but I did try to lose the weight that I felt sure was part of the problem. *If only I got skinny,* I'd tell myself, *I'll feel better. He'll love me again. I'll love me again.*

I'd try the latest fad diet—high protein, no carbs; pineapple for seven days; frozen diet dinners; complete restriction. Like most diets, they worked—for a while. But then I'd start my old, familiar, destructive eating patterns. I'd reach for my trio of favorite foods—the ice cream, the cheese, the peanut butter. They were my drugs, and I was an addict.

I know now what I didn't know then: when we pretend we are happy when we are not, when we bury painful experiences inside ourselves instead of confronting them, we end up hurting others—and ourselves most of all. But at that time in my life I was not aware of that important lesson, nor was I ready for it.

At that time, I thought that I had some kind of control over what I was doing; I believed that I could handle everything life dealt me, and that if I could just stop being as weak as I'd come to believe I was, I would be fine. I thought that losing weight was about self-control. I didn't have enough of it, I was told, and I told myself, but I knew this quality could only come from me so I didn't ask for any help. I kept my focus outside myself—on my beautiful, unique, wonderful daughters. I ignored myself, my body, my heart. I ignored what my gut was telling me: that I was unhappy, and that I was not being honored or respected. I used food to smother my desires. To take the place of dreaming and setting goals for myself. And I got very good at it.

If you've ever felt backed into an emotional corner and terrified of changing even one thing about your life, you probably understand this fear. It's not logical. It's not rational. But the fear of change surrounds you just the same. And it can feel much, much bigger than you.

Then, slowly, I risked really looking at myself. I stared at myself literally in the mirror and figuratively by allowing myself longer periods of self-focus. As uncomfortable as it was to see the differences, I started to compare the woman I was and the woman I felt that I ought to be. I examined what was still beneath the extra weight in my face, around my tummy, and at the top of my legs. I would stare long enough to imagine myself the way I used to be: an athletic, spirited young woman who wanted to be a teacher. Who loved a good run on a sunny, cool day. Who was the captain of a soccer team. Who swam competitively.

Where had that woman gone?

Where was she hiding?

I began to search.

The Turning Point

In the summer of 2000, I finally changed my life. I'll spare you the pitiful details of a bad marriage's ending, but suffice it to say that I finally began to question whether my marriage was truly tolerable and if, in fact, I was teaching my daughters to hide from their problems rather than try to solve them. I asked myself what kind of life I was truly modeling for my children. Was I teaching them that it is okay to let yourself go, to treat your body with disregard, to allow someone else's opinion of you to rule your life, to avoid and abandon your dreams and desires?

It was time for my girls and me to do the thing I had never thought I could do. I had to make a break from a marriage that had become toxic and from the life I was living. I didn't want my daughters to internalize the same sense of helplessness they saw me act out each day. I knew it was up to me to show them a new way to live, one based on taking care of myself and bringing health back to my life. I realize now this step took a tremendous amount of courage, but I was standing on the precipice and I was going to either fall or fly. I was gripped by the overwhelming desire to fly, to survive, to appear as my true self in this world.

Decision made, within months our home went up for sale, and the girls and I moved into a townhome nearby. I had done the unimaginable—broken out of hiding, removed myself from a bad situation, and created my own separate space. That first step seemed giant, but looking back, it was just one moment I needed to get to and through. And then we were out and moving forward. It was terrifying, but more than that, it was exhilarating and exciting.

In many ways this move was my first Start Here moment. It was the first of several baby steps that helped me reconnect to myself, to the inner strength that was always there but held locked up because of my own fears. I had a long way to go before I would feel completely emancipated and truly ready to embrace the lessons of those years, but I was on my way.

You probably can imagine how frightened I was to be suddenly on my own, needing to make a living, learning how to pay the bills and take care of the many details that go along with raising three young daughters. I had not really worked since I was in my early twenties. The whole job market had changed. My education seemed far away and almost useless. I felt beyond overwhelmed. I can still recall many moments when I felt nearly frozen with fear. Did I really leave him? Am I really the one in charge of myself and my daughters? But instead of retreating from these questions, instead of eating ice cream to smother my own voice, I actually began to answer them. Soon, I began to feel different. I began to feel stronger, capable, and trusting. Finally, finally, I was really in control of my own life! I felt safe. I was beginning to feel purposeful and powerful once again.

Within the safety of our own little townhome, I began to make changes in my diet. My daughters began to copy and follow these simple yet powerful dietary changes, the first of which was to try to stay away from my hidden foods—ice cream, peanut butter, and cheese in quantity! Instead I tried to eat more vegetables, fewer processed foods, and more protein. Quickly, I began to see positive changes in my health that even my doctor noticed and for which she congratulated me. And I lost weight. The dizziness and heart palpitations subsided. I felt more energetic. I slept more soundly. I was stunned at how easy it was to take back my health. Even with the smallest of changes, like putting the lid ON the peanut butter jar or NOT BUYING ice cream, my body was beginning to respond. It was dizzying stuff for a fat girl to now see and feel such powerful change.

I was beginning to feel so much better.

Coming Out of Hiding: The First Three Questions

Many of us use food to help us escape something that's wrong in our lives—it can be a huge, life-changing crisis, or it can be not-so-huge, everyday stress, fear, lack of satisfaction, lack of control, and countless other small feelings that grow into an all-consuming reality. We can also use food to block out feelings of inadequacy and self-loathing, feelings so old you can't even remember their original cause. But when food starts to be something that we hide ourselves behind, rather than enjoying it as a balanced part of a fulfilling life, simply recognizing the emotional association is the first and most important step toward turning things around.

In my work today, I like to make a distinction between food and nutrition. Food is simply something we indiscriminately push between our lips. Food has the power to break us down and destroy us, leaving us weak in the face of illness. Nutrition, on the other hand, is what we consume that feeds and sustains the body, and we should place it in a position of strength against what may confront us. The two are vastly different in my mind. When I think about food this way, it helps me stay committed to the latter and with optimal health fully in mind.

But back then, when I was trying to make this transition, I asked myself three tough questions:

1. Did I have the courage to face my reflection in the mirror?
2. Was that reflection really me?
3. If not, then why was I hiding?

When I got the courage to stand before the literal and physical mirror, I will admit that I was terrified. I didn't want to look at the overweight body standing before me. I didn't like the outline of the woman I saw. *In fact, I hated her!!*

Nonetheless, I did take that step and look at myself in the mirror in a new way. Doing so was a powerful signal to my psyche. Something inside me decided it was worth the pain and a second look to stare myself down. And what I saw was this: I had enclosed myself in layers of fat, which now hung on me like prison walls—meant to both protect me and punish me. I was not really made up of that extra weight. The real me was deep inside, hiding. I began to look at my relationship with food and noticed three things:

1. I ate not because I was hungry but because I was looking for comfort.
2. I protected myself through food.
3. I was now imprisoned by food that had become pounds and pounds of fat on my body, and I didn't know how to get out.

But I also realized that I was still a fighter. I just needed to believe it again. There I was, standing on my own, facing myself and my mistakes, and I didn't back down. I could survive this. No one was going to get the better of me again. Now all I had to do was re-create the fighter I knew I was. What kept hope alive for me was the knowledge that on the other side of this pain lay the promise of something much better—better health, more happiness, self-respect. I was also motivated by my kids. I knew my job as a mother was to be truthful and real—to show up every day as the strongest, brightest version of myself.

I now saw this prison of weight that kept me from myself with utmost clarity. I had let my favorite foods—ice cream, cheese, and peanut butter—hijack my relationship with myself. All that was left of me seemed to be the immovable walls of fat, the seemingly ever-present focus on what was around me—my then-husband and the problems in our marriage, my daughters and their needs, and of course the negative voice in my head. All of that kept me incarcerated. I no longer tasted the food; I no longer knew the excitement of a day not touched by shame. I no longer knew when my body felt hungry or full. It was as if I had lost all sense of my body. I had stopped taking care of myself. I had not stood up for myself. I had retreated into hiding. Somewhere along the way I had forgotten the simple fact that I could make my own choices.

I can reflect on that time as an incubation period in which, though I was dormant emotionally, I was still absorbing truths. It is often said that when people are under anesthesia for surgery, they can still hear and process what is said in the operating chamber. So though I felt anesthetized by food, I was still processing acutely all that happened—the good and the bad—and I was quietly gathering the strength to turn all those negatives into positives down the road.

Today I am in a much healthier place physically, mentally, and emotionally. I can even be thankful for the many ways I learned how to grow, thanks to the life I experienced with my first husband. If he had not tested me, I would not have known I was a warrior. I would not have found the qualities in myself that helped me get to where I am today and that saw me through a recent tragic episode in my life.

In 2012, my beloved second husband, Robert, died within three months of being diagnosed with cancer. Losing Bob was profoundly shocking and a terrible loss, the kind of trauma that could well have had the power to catapult me back to my old self-sabotaging/soothing patterns. But I didn't backtrack. My healthy eating is what grounds me; taking care of myself is what makes me strong, and I know that eating to cover up pain will only bring more pain. It was this attention to healthful nutrition and exercise that kept me from losing myself in my grief. I knew I could count on myself to survive. The hard-earned tools to do so were at my fingertips. It is a struggle to live without Bob, missing him every day as I do, but I have his gifts in my heart and I feel so proud to be able to carry them and him with me in what I do. This was true love as I had never experienced it.

Many life lessons are not learned, in fact, when times are good. They occur when the ground under your feet is unsteady. This is when you have to drill down into your core, searching for your true self. Not that I would ever wish to go back to the place where I started, but I do know now that without such tests, life is boring and leaves you emotionally shallow. I have become emotionally richer for all of the experiences I've had in my life, including the negative ones. I know how to be grateful for the complete range of life lessons handed to me.

I am a former fat girl. I was one of the invisible millions who are so threatened by the idea of change that we can't figure out how to stop eating—someone who, like you, was so fearful of altering even the slightest thing in my day that I stayed immobile.

But I came out of hiding, and now it's time for you to do so, too.

You Are Not Alone

Don't worry if you don't like what you see in the mirror. This journey is going to give you the power to change that image, once and for all, no matter how many times you've tried to take drastic steps forward before and felt like you failed. Your view of yourself can and will change.

You are one of millions trapped behind similar prison walls. I hear from so many readers and fans and friends that they, too, have found themselves far down an unhealthy road, only to come to some kind of turning point and know they must make a change. Sometimes these turning points are dramatic, sometimes they are mundane and subtle. And sometimes you see them only in your proverbial rearview mirror. But seeing them is the key, whenever it is you do so!

Consider Gloria, who had reached 260 pounds. As a young wife and mother of a four-year-old girl, her weight gain came from years of steady overeating. She and her husband were both obese and had been overweight when they married. Now she watched her daughter, who was a little plump, and thought, *What am I doing to her? What kind of life am I modeling for her?*

Gloria's turning point came when the family went on vacation. "We went on a trip to Florida. We were in the surf and some teenage boys made rude comments about me being fat. I wanted to die right there on the beach. Innocently playing in the soft curling surf was my four-year-old daughter, looking up at me as if I hung the moon and the stars! And then I noticed the tears running down her face."

For Gloria, her day of looking in the mirror was a result of once and for all taking responsibility not only for her own health but also for that of her daughter. Gloria opened her heart to that pain of the rude remarks, a powerfully emotional event, and had the courage to let the pain be the starting point of her journey. It was a tap on the shoulder to wake up and get busy changing her life. She received the message, did her personal homework, and manifested positive change in her life. She made the choice to fight rather than retreat.

You must discover your motivating moment yourself. Start here by asking yourself these three *dive inward* questions:

1. Do you have the courage to face your reflection in the mirror?
2. Is that reflection really you?
3. If not, then why are you hiding?

Now go to your journal and write down all that comes to mind. In my journal, I wrote these responses to those questions:

I am scared. I am terrified. But I know I can do it. I know somewhere inside me I have courage even though I am shaking like a leaf. I look outside the window at the vast winter sky and have to believe that this is the beginning of my journey, not the end of my life. The fat person in the mirror is not me. I am covered up. I am not made up of blubber and rolls of fat. I am inside somewhere, and I am going to find her.

I wrote down those words almost thirteen years ago. Since that time, my life has changed completely. And so can yours.

In the next chapter, you are going to take the answers to the questions you just asked yourself and build on them. One little step at a time, you are going to take down the prison walls. I promise, this *dive inward* is not complicated, but it will lead you directly to your pain and discomfort. You have to wrestle with this heart space because that's why you've been hiding—those feelings are what keep you imprisoned. Remember, too, that the ground must be unsteady under your feet for a little while before you can emerge from the pain, but it is a necessary unsteadiness that will yield a richness you can only imagine right now. Unsteadiness will actually make you feel totally alive. Stay the course!

The good news is that once you admit to yourself you *do* feel pain because you are overweight, you can look in the mirror knowing your reflection is not you. That reflection is only an altered version of you—

and you are now prepared to let the real you come out. It is as if you are standing in your fat self ready to unzip the layers of pounds, allowing your new self to emerge in a shining brilliance you have never seen before. When I realized this about myself, I felt incredible excitement—I was impatient to see this new version of me! And I am impatient to see the new version of you, too.

Your Journal: Look Inside Your Heart

⚘ To free yourself of your extra weight, you must recognize that you are, in fact, in a prison of sorts. You need to look inside yourself and acknowledge your pain. Once you've acknowledged pain, you must deal with it by removing it from your life, replacing it with forgiveness and hope, dreams and love. This allows healing. This allows you to move beyond the inner place that thinks of you as a fat person, so it's important to journal this valuable story for yourself.

On a blank sheet of paper in your journal, or on your computer, iPad, or smartphone, write a description of your prison (you can even speak it into a recorder or draw it if you prefer). Make a list of all the negative feelings about yourself that keep you imprisoned.

Throughout your dive inward journey, I will ask you to return to this place in your journal—to remind yourself of how you used to feel, to gauge how you are currently feeling, and to keep track of how you are changing. It may be painful the first time you do this, but you won't be able to move forward without establishing this important reference point. Don't wait for perfect words to appear. Just let the pen do the work while your heart empties out onto the page. Never correct what you write. Just write freely.

2

Step 1: Dive Inward

Mine was not a one-day uprising. My decision to leave my now ex-husband and rediscover, even re-embrace, my life took patience and perseverance. Yes, I had to admit that I was afraid to change—for months, for years. But finally, when I did have the courage to move into a home that was safe and all my own, I began to realize that along the way I had been making some important small changes just under the surface. In fact, in retrospect, I think it was those small shifts that made the biggest difference; they gave me the courage not only to leave that marriage but to find deep within me the power and courage to change the way I was living—forever.

Life is a mix of lessons and gifts—and it's up to us to find, nurture, and embrace both.

At the time, I was not ready for the life lessons that were embodied in my first marriage. Walled off and in pain, I let suffering define me. As I began to get back in touch with my inner strength and my gifts, I allowed the light to crack through the prison walls; then brick by brick, the walls around me began to crumble.

Then a powerful, positive force entered my life and helped me to see me: through his encouraging, loving, hopeful, and wise eyes, the real me began to take shape again. This force was Robert Kennedy, a man

I met at the school where I was teaching grade 1 and ultimately Robert's young daughter Chelsea. Becoming a teacher even at this late stage in my life gave me purpose and the means to support my daughters and myself at this highly uncertain time of my life. Robert not only believed in me and helped me to believe in myself again, he was also the man I eventually married, loved, and only recently said goodbye to when he sadly but courageously lost a blessedly brief encounter with lung and brain cancer.

Bob enabled me to see my life in terms of lessons: through his inspiration, I was able to transform the negative years behind me into positive momentum and motivation that got me where I am today.

I can't blame my ex-husband for how I was living, how I was eating, how I stopped exercising, or how I was taking care of myself. And I can't blame myself. Indeed, it's not a question of blame. Rather, it was a matter of asking myself a different set of questions that had nothing to do with blame, or being a victim, or looking for excuses. I knew in my heart that if I truly wanted to leave my marriage and change my life, it was up to me. And I would have to believe in *me* enough to overcome the powerlessness of not making changes. I also had to have the courage to face myself—my fears, my questions, and my self-doubts. I had been hiding too long and I could blame no one for that.

It became a question of responsibility to myself, to those I love and who love me.

So as you, too, begin to wrap your head around your desire to change, to lose weight, and to leave your pain and anguish behind, I ask you this question:

Do you know what's at stake?

By answering this question in this chapter, you will not only begin to find peace and clarity of mind; you will also begin to uncover those startling, amazing gifts that reside inside of you.

Your Journal

✐ What comes to mind when you think of the word *self-responsibility*? Do you take responsibility for your behaviors? Are you ready to take responsibility for how you feel? Do you tend to blame others in your life for the negative aspects of your life? Is there an old story that keeps defining your new life?

What's at Stake? Naming What Matters Most

When I look back at the experience of gaining so much weight and then losing it for good, I realize that getting in touch with my inner pain and suffering and giving myself permission to acknowledge how unhappy the extra weight was making me was the key. No diet was ever going to work in the long term without that realization. Sure, I knew how to lose a few pounds by restricting calories and cutting out desserts; I also knew how to lose a lot of weight by practically starving myself. But these and other methods always backfired. After a few weeks, I'd head back into the fridge or cupboard, looking for comfort. Why? Because I had never taken the time to really look inside of me to confront those long-unanswered questions. These are the ones that get right to the core of who you are, and they are going to help you shed the inner self-image of yourself as a fat person. They are going to get to the source of your pain. They are going to help you refind your gifts.

So let's get down to business.

Number one: Can you truly, honestly, and bravely figure out what's at stake for you?

Answering this question gets to the heart of why you want to lose weight.

Many diets begin by asking you to name a number of pounds you want to lose, or to identify your goals.

My strategy is a bit different: I want you to focus on what's *behind* your desire to lose weight.

Have you experienced a health crisis?

Is your weight limiting your life in a new, restrictive way?

Is your weight hurting someone you love?

Are you fed up with pretending that you are okay?

Are you no longer able or willing to lie to yourself and others to cover up how awful you really feel?

What's at stake for you is different from what was at stake for me. Indeed, identifying what's at stake is incredibly personal and unique. Not figuring this out now is what will keep you, and what kept me, from being fully able to embrace the three simple steps to this diet.

When I was trying to gather the gumption to lose all the weight I had gained over the course of my marriage, what was at stake at the first, most obvious level was the well-being of my daughters. I felt that living in the same house as their father was unhealthy, and it was my responsibility as a parent to provide a safe environment—physically, emotionally, and, yes, even financially. I couldn't do this, feeling as incapacitated as I did at that time. I knew weight loss—and health— had to happen for me to feel strong and resilient enough to be able to carve out a new life for me and my daughters.

Once I reached that point of clarity, all sorts of priorities began to shift.

After I made the decision to leave my first marriage, I could see clearly how I had not been taking care of myself. As many parents do, I took care of my children first; then I took care of my husband. I came last. To heal, I had to begin putting myself first, trusting that when I did so, I could be an even better parent to my three daughters. Nothing in life is more true than this: to take care of oneself is the purest sign of overall health. To be able to do it is the act of a true warrior. And once you determine what specifically is at stake for you, you will arrive at the same truth: you will finally be able to take care of yourself in a complete, whole way.

Gloria, whom I talked about earlier, was motivated to begin the process when she was struck by the image of her daughter's tears. Gloria had a glimpse of how her own health was making her four-year-old daughter grow up under an enormous shadow. Once in touch with how her obesity (and her husband's) was beginning to harm their daughter's health, she came to a dramatic realization: she had to change the way she was living both to survive to see her daughter grow up and to provide a better, healthier role model so that her daughter would not follow in her footsteps.

Everyone's reasons for positive changes have different triggers or motivations. Mark, a client who has found amazing success on the Start Here plan, told me that what got him started was the fact that he "had exploded from a 145-pound skinny guy in college to a 205-pound 'skinny-fat' guy as a 32-year-old professional adult. It was all in my belly."

As a pharmacist, he knew he needed to make some changes—or else, as he said,

I would find myself on blood pressure, cholesterol, and blood sugar medicines, just like "normal" middle-aged adults. Even though I was a pharmacist, I didn't really know where to get started with eating right. I grew up on a farm and healthy eating wasn't something I had learned. We ate a lot of meat and cheese. I never thought about portion sizes. That wasn't a problem until I left home and stopped moving around as much. But it took me years to figure out that my old eating habits were taking me down. When I finally changed the way I eat, I dropped from 205 to 158 pounds.

Answering the "what's at stake?" question usually leads to recognizing what matters most to us (those we love—our children, our parents, our partners, our pets) or some health situation that has become life-threatening.

For Helen, a thirty-four-year-old research scientist, it was realizing that the extra weight she was carrying had become a way of punishing herself.

I was in the midst of a divorce, caring for my ten-year-old daughter on my own. My husband had moved out and was not paying regular support. My stress level went through the roof. In one year, I gained fifty pounds. I had always been a bit overweight, but now, at only 5'3", I was officially obese according to my BMI. I'm a scientist; I know what stress does to the body. I also know what obesity causes: heart disease, among other things. For me, I had to stop because I realized I was going to kill myself. But I also realized that eating had become this twisted way of dealing with my fear of raising my daughter alone. I was terrified of being a single parent and the excess food was my way of pushing away the fear.

When Helen acknowledged her fear, she was able to begin the process of changing how she used food. She began to eat not for comfort but for nutrition.

What Are You Feeling?

I am going to ask you this question throughout the book. Being able to identify how you feel plays a huge role in your weight loss journey. If you feel sad, tired, lonely, or scared, these feelings can immediately set up obstacles to change; you have to remind yourself that feelings change and that *you are not your feelings.* Feelings are powerful indications of our reactions to what's around us, but they can change, and they don't have to overpower us. The first step to taking away their negative power is recognizing them.

> ## Your Journal
>
> ༄ Without too much thought, write down five to ten feelings you are experiencing right now as you are reading this book. List the feelings without judgment or criticism.

There are no right or wrong answers here. It's more about what's in your way and what matters to you. Some people even approach it more daringly: *What do I have to lose?*

Placing a name on what is at stake lends credibility to your decision making. How do you know what you are striving for if you can't name it? What is that "thing" you want, need, or must achieve? The name gives it purpose and direction, lending fire to the decisions that fall out of the simple task of naming "it." When you can name exactly what is at stake for you, then you can know for sure what you have to focus on. And that something becomes one of your concrete goals. If it is losing twenty pounds, then name it so. If it is wanting to fit into your college-day jeans (or a more modern-day version of them!), then name it so. If it is running a half marathon, as I did in 2010, then name it so. Suddenly out of all the murk will appear a clear and exact set of directions simply because you courageously named it.

Tosca's Journal

This is what I wrote in my journal when I first listed my feelings and my initial goals.

Scared

Alone

Determined

Courageous?

(Notice that I added a question mark! I wasn't yet sure that I had the courage, but I soon found out!)

Hopeful

Exhilarated

Insecure

Here is another excerpt from this early time in my life:

I need to do this for myself. I need to do this for my daughters. What kind of role model am I to three beautiful, strong, smart girls if I don't change and take better care of myself?

Are Your Basic Needs Being Met?

Are you emotionally safe in your life? Do you have access to healthy food? Do you have a safe home in which to live? Do you have loving support in your life? These may seem like obvious questions. You may even feel a bit offended by them—as if in posing these questions I am getting almost too personal, and prying into your privacy. However, these questions ask about basic human needs that we all should expect but cannot take for granted. Psychologist Abraham Maslow identified these needs in what he called the "hierarchy of needs," which I've adapted for the purposes of your dive inward.

Your Journal: Naming Your Needs

✒ If some of our basic human needs are not being met, then often taking even baby steps to change the way we live will feel too overwhelming. So indulge me and yourself for a minute by writing down your responses to these questions in your journal:

1. Do you have access to healthy, fresh foods to eat, water to drink, and air to breathe?
2. Do you sleep at night and wake feeling rested?
3. Is your digestive system working properly?
4. Can you rely on your body to move?
5. Do you have enough financial security through employment or other financial resources?
6. Do you feel in control of your health?
7. Do you have a safe place to live?
8. Do you have loving family and/or friends who are involved in your life?

If you responded "no" to more than two of these, then you probably feel too unsafe to take even baby steps toward change. I suggest you seek counseling, reach out to family members you trust, make an appointment with your doctor or health care practitioner—take concrete steps to create more safety and security in your life. In my mind the decision to seek counseling is one of the most courageous life-saving acts one can take. Many would not do so. You can. This is a rescue mission of enormous proportions and you will be able to celebrate your efforts.

What's Your Mindset? Shifting Everything

From the tiny window of your prison, it's often difficult—if not impossible—to see how vivid and vast the world outside can be. The view from inside is limited, and obscures the vastness of our potential, the startling gifts within us, and the beauty that surrounds us. When we dismantle the prison brick by brick, letting it crumble and disintegrate, our vision becomes clear and boundless. Soon the focus changes from the negative to the positive, where you are able to see a tiny crack of light, hope, and a way out.

This is the process that I went through when I began my life anew: I began chipping away at all that was keeping me feeling worthless, fat, and ugly.

This wasn't easy, but it was possible.

And I'm going to help you do the same.

There is a cliché that, though tired, is true: when a door closes, a window opens. From my earlier vantage point—a limited perspective obscured by my own dim view of life and pounds of excess fat—nothing seemed possible. Once I changed my view even just a little, I began to see possibilities. I knew I was a fighter, a survivor, and even a warrior. With that slim slice of hope I gave myself permission to take the smallest of steps. There I was. Standing. On my own. With the old life gone, I lifted one foot at a time in an unfamiliar direction guided only by my courage. I grasped at my freedom, finding opportunities in my teaching and interior design skills. One possibility at a time, I walked into a new life, gratified at every turn in my ability to believe in something I could not see but knew was there—survivor Tosca taking her rightful place.

Like most momentous, life-transforming decisions, I made changes slowly, piece by piece, letting myself feel safe as I made my moves. But after I identified what was at stake for me, I felt newly motivated.

One of the ways that I developed the courage and stamina to move forward in my life and change the way that I took care of my body was by shifting my attitude. Always an investigator and researcher, I had come upon the work of Carol Dweck, an interesting psychologist from Stanford who for years has been studying why some children seem more motivated and try harder in school, and some kids don't try as hard and just give up. She didn't believe that all the motivated kids were simply smarter. In fact, after years and years of research, she said the success of the kids who were motivated was not at all tied to intelligence but tied to their *attitude* toward intelligence. The more successful students had different underlying beliefs about intelligence that literally shaped their attitudes toward school, work, and, it turns out, life in general.

The kids who try hard and don't give up when they meet failure believe that their effort is what makes the difference. Dweck called this inner attitude toward our capability or potential to change "mindset." People who are easily dismayed by failure have a "fixed mindset"; those who believe that their effort matters have a "growth mindset"—they believe they can and will grow and change if they try.

Why did I find this concept of mindset so compelling? It meant that I needed to shift my mindset from a fixed view to one that would allow me to believe I could change—that it might take work and mistakes and even some setbacks, but with time and effort, I could not only lose the weight, I could change my entire life. And that's exactly what happened. This became so intoxicating an idea to me that I hardly was aware that I was losing weight, so intent was I on the mental shift I was making.

So let's see what your current mindset is and how we might nudge it in the direction of what I now call my new Start Here mindset.

Replacing What's Fixed with What Grows

My next challenge was recognizing the subtle but ever-present power that the negative voice—the *"you can't do anything"* voice inside of my head—had over me. It was what sabotaged my previous diets and in fact my entire life; what made me turn to food as a way to protect and comfort myself. This voice inside my head almost single-handedly kept me in prison. As Henry Ford famously said, "Whether you think you can or you can't, you are right." Isn't that the truth!

Of course, it didn't help matters that others reinforced my sense of powerlessness. Some people in my life still seemed intent on making me feel fat, ugly, and small, all at the same time. But I knew I couldn't blame anyone but myself for the state I was in if I wanted to change. Again, it was up to me to take responsibility.

Your Journal: Negative Voices

✺ Do you hear any negative voices in your head? What do these voices say?

Take a minute and write down any negative things you tell yourself. Next write down any negative things you recall other people in your life telling you.

Now put that list aside.

Going back to the work of Carol Dweck, you can indeed shift your mindset from one that is fixed and negative to a view that is growth-oriented and positive. I've adapted her ideas to create a three-step process that asks you first to identify any negative self-talk; second, to consciously shift your self-talk to a more positive, growth-oriented way of framing your attitude; and third, to practice and reinforce this new way of thinking.

First: Learn to recognize
the negative voices in your head.

A fixed mindset is discouraging and negative, and it will limit your belief that your life can change for the better. Do any of these phrases sound familiar?

1. You doubt your ability to change or succeed at weight loss.
2. If you hit a setback or obstacle, you conclude that you simply lack a special something. You suspect even your genetics are to blame.

3. You tend to blame others or find excuses for your mistakes or trouble.

4. If someone criticizes or questions you, you assume they are right, without questioning whether what they say is true or not. I call this "passive listening," in that you are not actively listening; rather, you behave as if you have already heard it all.

Second: Make a choice.

You can listen to these self-limiting ways of thinking about yourself, or you can choose to replace the negative with positive thoughts. Your Start Here mindset might sound like this:

1. "I'm not yet sure I can do this, but I think I can learn with time and effort."
2. "Most successful dieters and healthy people have failed along the way."
3. "If I don't try, I will definitely fail."
4. "If I don't take responsibility for my own life, I can't fix it."

Third: Realize that you have to keep making this choice until it becomes a habit, a new frame of mind.

1. Practice, practice, practice. When you consciously and mindfully hear yourself move from negative (fixed) to positive (growth) you will begin to change your thought patterns. Soon this will be your daily ritual and as simple as brushing your teeth—EASY!

By training yourself to have a new mindset, the way you think about yourself and the world will naturally begin to shift. But it doesn't happen all at once. You need to stay aware of your thoughts. Are they negative? Do they seem part of your new Start Here mindset or part of the old (fixed) mindset?

As I began to make these subtle yet powerful shifts in my own thinking, I also began to feel reconnected to some of the strength that I had slowly lost touch with living in a place that felt unsafe and in a body that I could barely recognize. When I began to replace negative, limiting thoughts with those that encouraged me to try, to grow, and to not be dissuaded by mistakes or obstacles, I felt suddenly liberated! I was beginning to dismantle the prison walls all around me. I was beginning to sense my own potential!

Yes, I could become strong—despite the years of abuse and despite my own negative thinking. This rebuilding would take time, but I now knew it was possible and it was up to me. What's more, the new faith I had in myself helped me feel deserving and even capable of creating something better.

When I look back at the energy it took to stay in my marriage and the energy it took to leave, I am surprised. The surprise comes from the realization that I was so strong. How did I not know this or acknowledge this strength earlier? Why did I let myself slip into submission? No matter how dim life got for me, I could always reach into a reservoir of light that kept me going. Something primitive in me wanted to survive, to make a mark and to succeed no matter what. And it is this transformation—the one that enabled me to embrace the extraordinary—that I wish to inspire in you.

We all have this strength inside of us. We all have gifts. You need to uncover *yours*, bring them out of hiding, and that is exactly what you are going to be doing next . . . *gently and easily.*

Your Gifts

As I took a closer look at how hidden in shame I'd become, I began to recognize and remember my gifts. What were the gifts that I needed to acknowledge? Years ago as a grade schooler I wrote for comfort. When my father suffered his first heart attack, I was a mere fourteen years old, but the planetary shift I experienced was more than I could bear. I placed those emotions on paper by writing an essay that would win first prize in a writing competition. I felt a surge of power in me as I was handed my winner's check, a feeling I can still summon today because what I knew for sure then and know for sure now is that *I* and only *I* did this.

Words have always been a source of comfort for me. They still are today. As you write down your truth in your journal, feel its weight, its reality. I still feel my truth even now. I recognized my strengths despite the stagnant life I was leading and used them, one by one, to lift me out into the light. Using one's talent is the most powerful way to emerge from a place of despair to a new place of purpose. Talent belongs to you and you alone. It is the only tool that can bring you fully into your place in this universe—the place you were meant to take. Four revelations crystallized my motivation:

I am a good mother.

I have a good brain.

I am not crazy.

I am a warrior and will survive.

These revelations gave me the courage to start here, to start now.

Your Journal: Finding Your Gifts

⚹ Each of you has gifts that are locked inside of you waiting to be rediscovered, and now it's time to refind them. This is possibly the most exciting part of your Start Here journey because you will finally have the ability to "see" yourself as never before. What you can accomplish will astound you. I am as excited for you as I was for myself when I went through my transformation. Life has never stopped giving back to me as a result. It will do just the same for you.

1. Close your eyes. What brings a feeling of joy to mind?
2. When was the last time you felt appreciated? What were you doing?
3. What makes you feel special?
4. How would you describe yourself as a child, before you became big or began overeating?
5. What gives you a feeling of support or love when you feel distressed or despairing in your current situation?

In many ways, these questions are leading you to one grounding question: What makes you, you? This is a critical piece of work that must be done as you are diving inward, and you are the only person who can do this. Allow yourself to fill up with the questions and to sit quietly as you reach for the answers. Chances are you probably already know what you want and have just been too afraid to say it out loud. Maybe you don't even think you are worthy of having a life. It's time to wind your story back to the days of hope you once had and reconnect with the joy of being you, making excuses for nothing. Life is not meant to be so difficult or sad. Write a new version of it that tells the story of a newly empowered you.

The Importance of Love and Belonging

✿ We are not meant to be alone, to live separately from our fellow human beings. As humans, we are essentially social and need to have the comfort and support of other people around us. This doesn't mean we have to be in constant contact with others, and it doesn't mean that living alone is a bad thing. What building a social life does mean, however, is that we build relationships with people who we trust, who we enjoy spending time with, who support us when we want to change things about our lives—for the better!

In this weight loss journey, you may feel yourself pulling away from certain people in your life. You may even feel some people pull away from you—especially those who feel uncomfortable or threatened by your healthful changes. Be aware of these tendencies, but stay connected. Stay in touch with those you love. You will need this support urgently now, as this first step may feel tentative. You may need much nurturing from others in the same place and on the same journey. Find a safe community. Join all the invisible millions who are connected worldwide at www.toscareno.com.

It's important to know that no matter how stuck you feel, you can change; you can remove the obstacles that have been in the way of your dreams and blocked your view of the real, *true you*—a you that has, until now, remained hidden under layers of extra pounds, and maybe even fear. That means you must open your prison door.

Allow what you read next to be your *permission to feel and be beautiful*, regardless of the size where you begin—ten pounds over where you'd like to be or 250 pounds.

It's time to come out of hiding.

It's time to inhabit your body.

It's time to take your place.

Gently. Easily. One step at a time.

3

Taking Your Place:

Getting Ready for Your Baby Steps

Congratulations! Now you've done some intense soul searching, and you've looked beyond the mirror to that inner place that houses your gifts and the true you. You have begun to silence the negative voices and replace them with an empowering new mindset that will support you as you ready yourself to take action.

Not that all of your inner work is over and done with. In fact, you are going to return to your feelings and your need for support again and again, as you troubleshoot obstacles and setbacks. Old patterns of behavior and negative, imprisoning thought cycles can take a while to tear down. This is to be expected. Don't panic if you slip up—that's why we spent the time we did on how to use your journal and other tips for taking care of your heart.

The main focus of this chapter is to help you prepare to take the next two steps of your Start Here plan. This chapter is not about taking action; instead, it's about getting yourself mentally and emotionally ready to start making changes, so read, relax, and take in the simplicity, the gentleness, and the ease of the two steps outlined below.

Removing Your Hidden Foods
and Moving a Little

These two baby steps—removing hidden foods and moving a little—reinforced my new mindset, awakened my body, and reset my system, leading me to lose weight gently but quickly. I didn't have to overthink what I ate. I didn't have to plan every snack and meal. I didn't have to join a gym. I kept my changes simple so that I could feel engaged in my own life again rather than starting a brand-new identity. One day at a time, I felt more confident. One day at a time, I realized that I had the tools to meet the inevitable obstacles that would stall or frighten me. All I had to do was take the tools out of the toolbox.

These steps are designed to be gentle and easy for anyone—whether you want to lose ten pounds, twenty, fifty, or a hundred. You will lose weight because I am going to show you how to remove certain foods that are messing with your metabolism and making you unable—until now—to lose the weight you wish.

You will start moving because I am going to show you familiar, comfortable ways to increase your level of physical activity so that your body comes back to life.

Even before you name your specific goal, I want you first to just read through the description of the two steps. It's important not to get ahead of yourself and rush to pin your entire life on some random number of pounds.

While you read about these steps and how they work, allow yourself some time to wrap your head around the simplicity of these actions. Accept that this way of eating and moving can lead to profound changes. Believe that you will achieve your goals and change your *life*. They are the two steps that I first used to change my life, and I believe they will change yours. They will not ask you to feel hungry, or even to join a gym. What they *will* ask you to do is to begin to feel yourself changing and find or rediscover a confidence in yourself and your abilities.

So before you put down the book to start trying out the tools, take a moment to really think about what I'm saying. I know you're in a hurry to start seeing changes in your life, but taking the time to live with this knowledge will reap enormous benefits and you will realize these benefits immediately.

The next two Start Here steps are *so* gentle and easy that at first you might just shake your head in disbelief. I really am asking you to do only two things:

1. Eat, but remove the "hidden food" that's sabotaging you.
2. Move *a little.*

You can't go through life denying yourself and feeling hungry all the time; that might work for a few weeks while you drop some weight, but the pounds will come back when the strain of denial finally breaks you down. This is why I don't ask you to make radical changes to your eating habits. Instead, when you realize what your hidden food is (and there may be more than one), remove it (or them), because you will see why these certain foods are at the root of your weight problem.

Remove Your Hidden Foods: A Quick Overview

Our hidden foods are those foods that literally make us fat. For me, it was peanut butter, ice cream, and cheese. These foods satisfied me most because I enjoyed their texture and could eat them in unlimited quantity. Or at least I felt that way. Somehow these foods conveyed comfort to me in the very moments when I needed them most. Many people who are overweight or obese have one, two, or three foods that account for 80 percent of their extra weight. Can it be so simple? It *is.*

For one man, whom I'll call Ben, the hidden food was Coca-Cola. The father of three, Ben went to bed night after night wearing sleep apnea gear due to his weight. He could no longer be intimate with his wife or wear normal sizes of clothing. His dreams lived in a slim man's world where running a half marathon and dressing in Armani suits were the norm. When he dropped that one food (yes, soda is a food!)—*just* this one step—he lost one hundred pounds in a year. How many Cokes had he been drinking? Twelve a day! But as soon as he removed the culprit, the rest of his diet—and his life—started to fall into place. In one year he went from being a highly medicated man to racing in a half marathon and wearing his designer suit. One year!!

My client Mandy zeroed in on her hidden food: mac and cheese. Mandy was eating mac and cheese with her kids at dinner, as an easy snack before lunch, and late at night when she was finally able to slow down and watch some TV. After turning thirty-eight and contemplating whether or not she could go to her twentieth high school reunion, she realized that she couldn't stand looking at herself anymore. In twenty years, she had gone from a size 10 to a size 18. She felt tired all the time, her skin was rough and patchy, and she had to shop in the plus-size area of department stores. Finally she had had enough.

At first, she was nervous about diving inward and asking herself some tough questions. She felt enormous shame about having gained weight, was embarrassed to go out with her friends, and was terrified of seeing her entire high school class. I helped to guide her as she began to look at how her mindset was holding her back. After getting in touch with the spirited girl she used to be, Mandy was ready to identify her hidden food—the mac and cheese was the glaring culprit! Once she removed it from her diet, she felt very clearheaded and began to cue into her body in a new way, losing almost ten pounds over two months. Her basic diet had not been all that bad. She needed to reduce her portion sizes and replace the mac and cheese with tasty grilled chicken salads and other fresh foods. And in less than four months, she dropped twenty pounds. She felt better than she had in years!

Karin, a former model, had put on twenty pounds over the ten years in which she had two daughters—ten pounds per pregnancy. At 5′6″, she had always been athletic and weighed about 125, more or less. By age forty-two, she was hovering around 150. Her hidden food? White wine. She loved the taste, it helped her relax, and she felt it was "safe"—it wasn't like she had a drinking problem. A week after she removed the white wine from her diet, she lost five pounds. By the next month, she'd lost ten.

But Karin's dive inward had revealed some important life lessons: as a former model, she had a very ambivalent relationship with food. She loved it; she hated it. As a young girl and woman she was told she was "naturally thin," but as soon as she hit twenty-five, she couldn't control her eating. She binged when she was alone: eating cartons of no-fat ice cream and frozen yogurt, and then forcing herself to throw up. She would then practically starve herself for days, eating only celery sticks and wheat thins.

When she got married and had her first child, Karin's relationship with food settled down a bit. She was very healthy when she was pregnant and nursing, and when her daughters were young. But slowly, she began to rely on a glass of white wine—or two, or three—to relax in the evening.

By the time she reached my door, so to speak, Karin believed that to stay thin, she had to avoid most foods, so she was dumbfounded to realize that she had gained twenty pounds simply by drinking wine. She also thought that her wine habit was under control. For Karin, simply removing her hidden food was not enough; she had to do a lot more processing of her body image and other misconceptions about her identity before she could trust herself again and develop a healthy relationship with food.

I am happy to say that after two years, Karin has successfully quit her white wine habit, eats as healthy as her now-teenage daughters, and, most important, knows that she can take care of herself.

Our hidden foods are typically fatty, salty, starchy, or sweet. Sometimes they contain fat, salt, and sugar—all at once! But what's "hidden" about the food isn't that it's in disguise; what's hidden is that we are eating it unconsciously, without really thinking or paying attention. This kind of eating is similar to eating with wild abandon, pretending the endless mouthfuls are nothing, as if we've become addicted to the food—and in most cases, we have.

So in step 2, I am asking you a simple question: "What is the one food that you can't live without?"

The answer to that question—the first thing or couple of things that come to mind—is most likely your hidden food.

But don't jump ahead. You may not yet know what your hidden food is. Keep reading. Soon, you will gain clarity. And I promise you this: when you remove that one food (or two or three, as was the case with me), you are taking your first baby step toward losing weight and saving your life. With this one step, you are then able to gently clean and balance your body's system, replace your hidden food with other things that taste good and fill you up, which then enables you to begin to speed up your weight loss. With just this one step, you will feel lighter, cleaner, and more clearheaded than you have in years.

If you find yourself feeling good without your hidden food, you can choose to take another small step—and lose more weight even more quickly—by removing other foods—hidden *culprits*—masquerading in your meals and snacks, foods that are getting in your way of losing weight even faster, but *also* interfering with how you *feel* physically and emotionally.

Once you feel more stable and trusting of yourself, you will "replate" your food, taking the bad out of hiding and replacing it with foods that are delicious and healthy, and that maximize your weight loss.

Your breakfast options are delicious—Apple Cinnamon Oatmeal, Breakfast Sausage, Goat Cheese and Chive Omelet, and even pancakes! Lunch and dinner are even more tasty—choices include Hawaiian Chicken Burgers, Sloppy Joes, Spicy Shrimp and Sausage Gumbo, and corned beef and cabbage. You can even enjoy a Taco Night!

You will not ever feel deprived. You will not ever feel hungry. You will not only enjoy these wonderful, tasty, easy recipes, but you will also gently expand your repertoire of foods so that beans become familiar, arugula salad a must-have at least once a week, and almonds and cashews your new best friends. Removing your hidden food will anchor a new way of eating that will become as natural as sand on the beach!

Why am I reminding you of all this? So you don't panic. So you don't slam the book shut and devour a dose of your favorite comfort food. So you realize that you are in good hands—mine and your own. You will redefine your relationship with food as you eat. The more your body takes in the good and leaves out the bad, the better you will feel. This good, clean feeling will motivate you and sustain you.

Moving a Little

In step 3 of your Start Here plan, I ask you to move . . . *a little*. I don't ask you to join a gym, start jogging, or invest in a treadmill. Sure, those exercise options are out there. But what you are going to do is simply go from not moving . . . to moving a little. That's it.

Here's how this simple approach to exercise works. I offer you two lists to choose from: the first lists twenty-five everyday activities and the second, twenty-five basic, easy movements. Both lists are likely to be chock-full of activities and movements that most of us do each day without thinking about them—from sweeping floors, to washing out cupboards, to putting away laundry piece by piece. These activities are meant simply to welcome you to a new way of approaching your day, gradually and steadily increasing your amount of physical activity. When you begin to integrate even the simplest movements, you will start to feel more flexible and literally more able to move.

I hear from many people beginning the Start Here plan that they can barely imagine moving, never mind actually putting one foot in front of the other. Which is why these activities are so doable. Walking your neighborhood? Doing a bit of gardening? Playing with your kids? Washing your car? You can and you will! And best of all, you will learn how to do these everyday activities in a way that will help you lose weight and become more fit in the process.

Connie was over three hundred pounds when she found this program. For over ten years, she had become so sedentary that the only movement she could manage each day was getting herself out of bed, to the bathroom, and then resettled in her favorite recliner. She depended on her sister, with whom she lived, to make her meals, do her laundry, and take care of all other aspects of her life.

At only forty-two years old, Connie was overwhelmed with sadness and self-disgust. After removing her hidden foods (in Connie's case, this was a bit complicated—not only did her diet consist of sugary packaged baked goods, but the size of her portions was enormous), she was terrified to begin step 3. After much back-and-forth, we decided that she should simply try getting up and out of her chair and walking to and from her bedroom. Then she added walks around the house. After a couple of weeks, Connie was able to walk to the end of her driveway and back—*without assistance*. For Connie this was an amazing milestone, one that helped her to begin making movement a regular part of her life.

Whatever you can do now, wherever you find yourself, you will discover ways to incorporate movement into each ordinary, otherwise crazy-busy day. We start small—fifteen to twenty minutes of walking around the supermarket, or a few minutes of lifting your legs, one at a time, while sitting on the edge of your sofa. After a few days, you will learn how to gradually build up to twenty to thirty minutes of movement—maybe that means thirty minutes of vacuuming while holding in your belly; maybe that means combining fifteen minutes of pulling weeds with fifteen minutes of wiping down the refrigerator or cleaning the bathtub. That's it. The idea is to incorporate movement into activities you *already* do—just do them smarter. Not to mention, just imagine how many things you'll tick off your to-do list!

These two steps—remove your hidden food and move a little—will support your secret strengths and help you lose the weight that's strangling your life and keeping you locked up. You will learn how to remove the foods that are making you fat and start to move *a little*, so you feel alive once more.

I'm not a trainer or fanatic who is going to act tough, bark orders, and insist you go through life as if it were a boot camp, readying you for battle. My approach is different. I am going to nourish you, support you, and help you connect to that place you have inside—those gifts that make you, you.

But remember: you will

- never feel hungry
- lose at least one to two pounds per week
- feel lighter, more energetic, and clearheaded than you ever have before
- regain purpose and desire in a life worth living

You may feel afraid; you may think that anything to do with food is scary. And even thinking about changing our relationship to food is scary, no doubt about it. But your life is about to change.

You are going to forgive yourself once and for all so that you can finally lose the weight that has been holding you back from your *real* life.

You are about to take a momentous step that is surprisingly gentle and easy. The two steps are not complicated and they are so good for your body.

Over the next days, weeks, and months, you will be caring for yourself in a way that you will never get from counting calories or having someone scream at you to "lose weight." I understand these all-important first steps better than anyone, because I have been the fat person wanting desperately to be done with diets. The only way to accomplish this is to make the changes feel as normal as brushing your teeth—to make them as simple as baby steps.

Tosca's Journal

I took a wrong turn today. I not only ate dessert for breakfast (leftover birthday cake) I then tried to starve myself the rest of the day. Well that didn't work. It never works. I feel miserable. I have a headache. I just need to go to bed. Tomorrow is another day.

Building Your Foundation

The Start Here plan is simple and straightforward—you remove the foods that are sabotaging you and you move a little. For this simplicity to work, it's important to give yourself opportunities to bolster your confidence, troubleshoot obstacles, and forgive yourself if you slip up. Be honest with yourself. Don't try to push away your fears, discomfort, or any other sign that you are encountering difficulty. Instead, use these telltale signals that your brain and body are giving you. Stay open to all your thoughts and feelings so that you know what you are experiencing. And trust that you are building the tools to meet these obstacles head-on.

Each step takes you in the direction of your goal. Every word is meant for you to get closer to a new you with no wrong turns. Here are five important things to keep in mind as you move forward:

- *Reach for your support.* You don't have to—nor should you—go it alone. I encourage you to enlist a buddy to join you in the program, reach out to a sympathetic ear, or log on to www.toscareno .com for support from my existing 200,000-member "Kitchen Table" online forum or the fast-growing "Start Here" support forum.

- *No one is perfect.* You give everyone else around you a break; do yourself the same favor! Every time you check in with yourself, and give yourself support instead of an internal bash, you reinforce your new commitment toward your goal.

- *Keep your goals simple.* When it comes to setting goals, you want to challenge yourself, but not so much that you feel overwhelmed. It's important to strike a balance between raising the bar but ensuring that you have the physical energy, emotional support, and mental clarity to make realistic, attainable goals. These may change from day to day, week to week, month to month. Goals are not meant to be laws written in stone, but rather are guidelines that work to motivate and encourage you. By keeping your eye on the three steps of the Start Here diet, you can keep your goals simple while also feeling like you are making good, steady progress.

- *Reward yourself.* Just as it is crucial not to harbor negative or judgmental attitudes or thoughts about yourself, so is it equally important to reward yourself—physically, mentally, or emotionally. What do I mean by this?

  - Go to a movie.
  - Download a new novel on your e-reader.
  - Call a friend and get your nails done.
  - Get a massage.

Start Here is all about cherishing the you who is so wonderful!

- *Stay present.* When you stay focused on today, you can be more alert to what is really happening in your body and how you are feeling. Yes, I want you to have goals to shoot for—one-week goals, one-month goals, six-month goals, and forever goals. But it's equally important to *just focus on this step, now; this step, today.* Use your journal to keep track of your feelings, what you're eating, what you're doing. This is your journey, and your journal is a record of this magnificent time in your life!

Your Journal: A Quick Exercise

⅋ For each of the bulleted items above, write a few sentences that come to mind:

- Who in your life is able to *support you*? Make a list of people who love and respect you.
- *Forgive yourself* for the past diets that have failed and the days ahead when you may reach for your hidden foods in a moment of panic and distress.
- Remind yourself of your goals—near or far—and let them motivate you.
- How are you going to *reward yourself*? Make a list of enjoyable ways to reward yourself for all the work you have accomplished.
- What helps you *stay present*? Taking a walk in the evening? Praying? Free-writing in your journal? Meditating? Make a list of four or five things that you can do to create a calm atmosphere that allows you to focus and be still.

Creating Realistic Goals

Your goals are meant to mark the milestones along the way as you progress from Fat Person, as I once was, to New You, which you soon will be. However, goals can only be successful if they are reasonable. No one ever ran a marathon without running a few 5Ks first. Step by step is the way to success. As you move along, check in with yourself weekly. How are you doing? Measure it, mark it, celebrate it—but stay in touch with *you* as you move forward. This is exciting and it's progress!

When I was beginning this process, I started by removing my hidden foods—the ice cream, cheese, and peanut butter. That's all I could do for about a month. Then, as my body adjusted and I began to feel more clearheaded and energetic, I wanted to move. I began with swimming. I had been a competitive swimmer when I was a teenager, and getting in the water again—even if I didn't yet like my shape—made me feel light. I began slowly. Lap by lap. I would swim for fifteen minutes—which felt like an eternity!

But as the weeks and months passed, I could swim twenty minutes, then thirty minutes. My confidence began to increase. As soon as it was summer, I felt like I was ready to add in fast walking. Here's a snippet from my journal at the time.

> *I feel exhausted today but also exhilarated! I swam 15 laps and even had energy left over to take a walk with the girls! I'm going to the mall this weekend and buy myself a new pair of jeans and a sexy top!*

Near and Far Goals

The Start Here plan is meant to last you a lifetime. But to begin, all I want you to do is think about week 1.

For seven days, you are going to remove one hidden food. That's it.

Once you determine what food you want to remove, which you will do in the next chapter, you'll then decide *how* to begin to move a little.

You will see, I am not asking you to start weight lifting, doing jumping jacks, or running around the block. I am asking you to incorporate just fifteen to twenty minutes of movement into each day.

That's it.

After you have done these two steps for seven days, you will be able to determine your two sets of goals:

- Near goals
- Far goals

Your *near goals* are what you want *to do* in weeks 2 through 4.

- Do you simply want to focus on removing one hidden food for four weeks straight and see where that leads?
- Or do you want to try going cold turkey and remove two or three hidden foods all at once?
- What kind of movement do you want to try to incorporate?
- How much time per day and per week can you commit to?

Ask yourself what you want to do about food and about movement. Those are the parameters of your near goals.

Your *far goals* are where you would like to end up:

- How much weight would you like to lose?
- Do you want to be able to play with your kids in the yard or park?
- Do you want to be able to walk your daughter down the aisle?
- Do you want to live to see your first grandchild?
- Do you want to beat a diagnosis of type 2 diabetes?

Far goals are aspirations. They are meant to be end goals, achievements that will happen over time.

Near goals are meant to keep you in the present, focused on putting one foot in front of the other so that you don't get intimidated or overwhelmed by the bigger picture. This is why I encourage people to create realistic goals on a week-to-week basis. Use your journal to write down your goals and keep revising them daily or weekly—whatever feels most natural to you. These first three weeks are huge, hard, and very intimidating—not because of their complexity, but because they ask you to make small changes that will more than likely bring uncomfortable feelings to the surface.

Again, by keeping your focus on your near goals, with the far goals off in the distance, you give yourself permission to work through difficult feelings—and more than likely in ways that are successful.

Your Journal:
Check In with Your Feelings and Mindset

✎ Are you feeling lonely today? This is so common! It's easy for those of us inside the prison walls to feel attacked and separated from the pack. But take a minute or two or twenty and reach out to someone you care about. Don't even think about sharing your feelings; instead, start by asking your friend, sister, uncle, or co-worker how they are feeling. By extending this compassion, you will feel better. You may also invite your friend or loved one to ask the same question of you: How are you feeling today? When you share how you are doing, you give yourself the opportunity to acknowledge your feelings, accept them, and then move on. Once you begin to live outside of yourself, bringing your particular brand of joy to the world, it becomes so gratifying you won't be able to stop. Keep on giving love and you will receive it in vast quantities.

When the logistics of life interfere with your steps, what small tweaks can help you keep going? A huge roadblock for many people is thinking that making changes is just too big for them to handle. Instead of doing nothing and sticking with your bad habits, make a small change—maybe it's a 5 percent change; maybe it's a 10 percent change. As we move ahead together, look for opportunities to make small changes. Ask yourself, "What little thing can I do today that gets me 5 percent closer to my goal?"

In chapter 9, you'll learn many strategies to manage roadblocks and other ways that good eating can get interrupted by life—vacations, parties, holidays. But for now, as you are preparing yourself to identify and then remove your hidden foods, it's important to keep in mind that you can set your own pace. You can take out one food at a time. You can go cold turkey. You can try taking out one food and then another. This is a simple plan that works but it also offers you options and flexibility.

In the next chapter, you will be ready to take action. After all of the inner work you did with your dive inward, as well as the mental preparation and goal setting you accomplished in this chapter, you are ready to take your next baby step! How awesome is that?!

PART TWO

Losing Weight and Regaining Yourself

4

Step 2:

Remove Your Hidden Food

Let me ask you a simple but powerful question: *What are the one or two foods that you think you cannot live without?*

In my experience, it's not a dozen foods that keep us from losing weight, but one, two, or three old standbys that keep us at our less-than-ideal weight.

I call the foods that sabotage us "hidden foods" because they are often not the food that we eat during meals, but rather food we may eat incidentally, or the food *inside* the food that we think is otherwise healthy to eat. Your hidden foods can also be a question of quantity: a roll with dinner every once in a while is not necessarily bad, but if you eat starchy white breads, rolls, and crackers with every meal, every day, then the quantity of such a powerful food can indeed disrupt your entire metabolism.

If your hidden food *is* something on your dinner plate, it is likely that you don't realize the power of that food to keep your weight high. Let's be honest. It is not just about the hidden food but about how much of that food you are consuming. I could sit all night with a gallon of ice cream and kill it before I went to bed. That is a lot of ice cream! Quantity matters as much as quality.

What's your hidden food? The answer to this question may not be immediately apparent. It may take some thinking and some honest soul-searching. But then again, it may be really obvious—the giant elephant in the room. It may not even be one food but a couple or a few.

I knew a woman who went to bed every night with a tray of brownies under her bed. When she woke each morning the tray was empty. This was her hidden food and her nemesis. Another person ate bacon with virtually every meal—she indulged in it with her eggs, as you might expect, but also coupled it with cookies after a meal! Four hundred and ten pounds later she was heading for a health disaster.

As soon as you identify your hidden food(s), you are halfway to completing step 2 of your Start Here plan.

When I began to pay attention to what I was eating, it became clear that these three foods—ice cream, peanut butter, and cheese—were the source of most of my extra calories. The rest of the day, I ate relatively healthy. I was a good cook and fixed homemade meals for my family—I didn't use a lot of fat or sugar. My head seemed to be in the right place for the hours of the day that I was in front of my family, and I badly wanted to be the best mother I could be. But when on my own, I reached for my favorites because I justified my earlier efforts as deserving of a reward. I saw those foods as treats that I could eat because I had worked so hard during the rest of the day (both to eat the right things and also to keep it all together).

A lot of people (me included!) rationalize that eating a half carton of ice cream for dessert is offset by all the veggies on the dinner plate, or that eating a full-size bag of dark chocolate M&Ms is okay because dark chocolate is the kind that's good for you. But as time went on, and I saw my shape fade away in the mirror, my body hidden under baggy clothes, I looked at my healthy family and knew I was doing something different. When I was able to look plainly at how and what I was eating, I realized that my hidden foods were indeed sabotaging me. They were the cause of the extra pounds. They were the source of the unevenness in my moods and what was disrupting my metabolism.

> ## Your Journal: Where Are You Eating?
>
> ✒ If your meals are more or less healthy, with normal-size portions, then your hidden food may not be on your plate. Do a quick inventory to see where you keep what you eat throughout the day:
>
> > Your cabinets
> > Your desk drawers
> > Your car
> > Your refrigerator
> > Your purse or briefcase
> > Your bedside table
> > Your trash container
>
> Food wrappers and empty cups or containers are probably hiding in plain sight. These could be clues to your hidden foods.

How to Look for Your Hidden Foods

If you're looking at your daily habits and aren't sure how to find the ones that are detrimental to your life, you need to be honest with yourself about what you're eating throughout the day, and then check the nutritional value of that food. Is it made up of calories that your body will use? Is it on the list of common hidden foods (See "What Is Your Hidden Food?")? If you determine that your hidden food is, indeed, useful to your body, then maybe it's the amount you are eating that is causing the weight problem.

If your hidden food is in the empty-calorie category (see "Empty

Calories That Make Us Fat"), then you need to make a decision: Is it really worth eating? Again, this matters because certain foods, such as spaghetti and meatballs or even diet soda, appear healthy, but eating them in large quantity is damaging to health and weight loss goals. Even peanut butter, a seemingly healthy food made from nuts, is not so healthy if consumed by the shovelful, as I once did. If this hidden food is the source of your weight problem—if it triggers overeating *and* gets stored as fat—then it is working against you. I would also like to suggest that some of us eat for taste alone—sweet, salty, savory— indulging for that fact alone and never to good result. Taste is itself a partial driver but nutritional satiation is the pinnacle we must strive to reach.

As you make small changes to the way you eat and live every day, you may have to abandon these hidden foods because they are really trigger foods that launch you into an eating frenzy. Even today I must carefully measure these foods if I plan to eat them; otherwise, I may feel triggered to eat them without limit. Each of you will have to deter- mine whether these hidden/trigger foods will reappear in your diet later on. This may be a question of whether eating a certain food is worth it. Will it trigger you to lose control? Can you have a bite or two of chocolate birthday cake at a friend's office party and not rush home to dive into a candy bar or half a pint of ice cream because "it's too late now"?

Whether or not you can ever reintroduce your hidden foods is a deeply personal question, and only you can know the answer. You may reach a point where you feel so balanced that you can enjoy one of your hidden foods without setting off a domino effect; on the other hand, you may want to be safe rather than sorry. Let's return to this question as we move through the plan. Ultimately, it's up to you to decide how much of that hidden food you want to be eating.

Can it be a little scary to be honest with yourself this way? Sure—but it can also be empowering. Where previously you may not have known *what* kept you above your preferred weight, now you'll *know.* Now the information will be in *your hands,* and that's a powerful thing.

Finding your hidden food can be a bit tricky.

Let me share with you a couple of stories from clients who identified and then removed their hidden foods and nothing else—with amazing results.

As a young woman, Toby was slender and could eat whatever she wanted. She was never very active, but didn't have to worry about her weight. When her friends were off playing soccer and basketball, Toby was content to hang out after school and watch TV. By the end of high school, she'd put on some extra weight—maybe ten pounds—but since she was tall (5′9″), the pounds seemed to distribute evenly and she felt okay with how she looked. After finishing a two-year associates' degree, with a plan to go into nursing, Toby and her boyfriend decided to get married. Quickly thereafter, Toby got pregnant, and gained about seventy-five pounds during her pregnancy. She wasn't worried. She was a big woman and felt comfortable with the extra weight, believing that she was creating a strong, healthy child.

When her son Tyler was born, Toby lost about fifteen of the seventy-five pounds. But in the months and years following, she put back the fifteen pounds, plus a few more. By the time she was twenty-nine, she weighed almost 290 pounds.

What was Toby's hidden food? Mayonnaise. She added full-fat mayonnaise to every dish she prepared—from deli meat sandwiches to tuna and macaroni casseroles to mashed potatoes and burgers, meat loaf and fish tacos. Toby so loved the taste of mayonnaise, she invented ways to incorporate it into dishes, snacks, and even desserts. She ate pretzels and chips with mayonnaise dip; she ate fruit cake made with mayonnaise. She even created a fruit smoothie with mayonnaise.

Do you know what's in most popular brands of mayonnaise? Oil, egg yolk, and sugar. But it's the oil that contains the most lethal ingredient: hydrogenated fat.

Compounding the damage of the mayo were some of the high trigger foods she paired with it: deli meats, burgers, and starchy potatoes. These foods in isolation may not be totally bad, but in high quantities and alongside mayonnaise, they become fat grenades, detonating your body's natural order.

Amazingly, when Toby identified her hidden food and removed it—not completely but *most of the time*—she immediately lost weight quickly and safely. She never felt hungry, and she didn't change her level of activity. In two weeks, she had lost eight pounds; in two months, she'd lost twenty-five pounds; and in one year, she'd lost ninety pounds.

Angela's story is a bit different. She had always been a chubby kid. Her mother was chubby. Her grandmother was chubby. Her maternal aunts were chubby. The women in the family were also short, with no one reaching beyond 5'3". Throughout her young adult life and twenties, she'd probably tried twenty different diets, and watched in hope and frustration as her weight went up and down, up and down—usually ending up, once again. By the time she was in her thirties, Angela was both a diet pro and a cynic: she no longer trusted any diet, and did not believe that weight loss could be maintained.

It wasn't until Angela took a hard look at her eating habits that she was able to make a real breakthrough. When she asked herself what food she could not live without, the answer was clear: bread. Finally, she seemed ready to clean up and simplify her life and end her misery.

How bad could bread be? you may wonder. Bread has no fat, right? Most breads are indeed low in fat. But what they are often hiding is what I call their "puff factor"—the starchy, spongy quality that makes white bread so soft and satisfying to eat. In fact, if you ask most people what it is about bread that they love, they typically refer to bread's texture, or its smell. So in the case of bread, it's not even about the taste; it's about how bread *feels*.

When Angela looked at how her family ate—her mother, aunts, and grandmother—she saw how bread was always positioned as the star of the meal or snack:

- Breakfast featured toast or English muffins.
- Lunch was a big sandwich on fluffy white bread.
- At dinner a basket of dinner rolls sat in the center of the table.

Everyone began the meal with a roll and ate at least one more during the meal.

We will get into the way your body reacts to certain foods later on, but for now suffice it to say that after years of overreliance on bread in building her breakfast, lunch, and dinner plates, Angela's body was not only addicted to bread, it was no longer able to fully metabolize, or digest, it. The result? On Angela's body, the bread became fat.

When I met Angela she was 5′2½″ and weighed 175 pounds. When she identified and cut out bread as her hidden food, she lost twenty-five pounds in six months. She was elated.

Once Angela added physical activity to her weekly routine, she began to lose even more weight, finally reaching her ideal weight of 137. In the process, she also gained lean muscle, which made her body stronger and more efficient. She now looks slender, but even more important, she has changed the way her body metabolizes food. The best news? Angela can enjoy bread and rolls every once in a while without triggering overeating. Even better news is that Angela is healthy!

Every body is different and reacts differently to certain foods. Your hidden food, like Angela's, may be bread; but your best friend may be able to eat bread and sweets without feeling compelled to eat them with abandon. What's crucial is learning to pay attention to how your body reacts to certain foods: if you feel logy, slow, or agitated after a meal that is loaded with starchy carbs like pasta or potatoes, that's a very good sign that you are *reactive* to white flour-based foods.

Of course, hidden food doesn't affect only women and men with a great deal of weight to lose. In many cases, a hidden food can be the thing that prevents someone from losing those last dreaded ten pounds. Gary had been an athlete all his life. But after college, life happened. As he describes it:

I had a wife, kids, and a job. A couple of decades later and I found myself in the worst shape of my life. I developed a weight lifting habit in college as a means of relaxation that I'd kept, but any muscle I'd built over the years was, by age 43, covered in fat. I wasn't obese by any means but I wasn't my old self . . . my fit self.

My turning point came when my oldest son got married. Being fitted for a tux was eye-opening. I had no idea my waist had gotten that big. And then came the wedding photos. I was shocked. At what point in my life did I become Tony Soprano? Rather than wait for the turn of the New Year, which I could have easily done . . . and was tempted to do, I decided to take immediate action.

After just a couple of weeks I began to think differently about the things I put into my body. Whereas I used to gobble, I now began to eat more slowly, thinking about the foods I put in my mouth. Now I'll be the first to admit I wasn't perfect. My demon? Beer. I'm a beer snob I'll readily admit. I like my beers strong, flavorful, and full of calories. I don't do light beers. So giving up beer entirely, while recommended, simply wasn't an option. So I cut back. I adopted a "never if I have to work the next day" rule which, essentially, cut me back to just two days a week. But this was far and away my biggest diet challenge.

Gary lost his ten pounds and has kept them off for the past five years! And because he is now in better physical shape, increasing his lean muscle and decreasing his fat, he also can enjoy a beer every now and then.

But let me give you fair warning: reintroducing your hidden foods can be dangerous. You need to make sure you can read your own body's signals and therefore trust your ability to monitor your foods. Exercise and building muscle is a wonderful way to manage reactiveness to trigger foods, but sometimes even being in good shape is not enough to buffer a domino-like effect. So for the first four to six weeks of step 2, it's best to simply remove your hidden foods.

Empty Calories That Make Us Fat

✻ How can you identify foods that pack a lot of calories but offer zero nutrition? Most packaged baked goods, sugary cereals, even "enriched" bread products contain a blend of calories that offers minimal substantive nutrition—what I call empty calories. Pretzels, chips, and Goldfish fall into this category. Why is this dangerous? Because these foods are designed to be eaten quickly and never fill you up! Because they lack a balance of protein, complex carbs, and healthy fat, your body does not recognize them as real food. So what happens? The calories are rerouted to fat, and worst of all, you remain hungry!

Soda or pop is another huge calorie-dense food that offers no nutrition. Remember the man who was drinking thousands of calories of Coke every day? Clearly he did not understand how dramatic the impact of seemingly harmless eating is. We know we're not supposed to eat fried food every day, but what's wrong with peanut butter? Or a box of spaghetti with meatballs every day? It's very important to think about the food you are eating; if it's not "grown in nature," then make sure you check its label. Once you identify your hidden foods and begin to eat more cleanly (i.e., dropping the packaged and processed options and relying instead on fresh foods), then you will probably lessen the chances of unwittingly eating empty calories. But until this is second nature, beware!

> ## *Tosca's Journal*
>
> *Ice cream, peanut butter, and cheese. The triumvirate of terrible foods—they make me feel terrible and look terrible. Will I miss them? I guess so . . . for a while.*

What Is Your Hidden Food?

If you've been thinking about this question since I posed it earlier, you may already know your primary hidden food.

Here is a list of very common hidden food culprits:

Dairy

Cheese

Dips

Ice cream

Sour cream

Butter

Starchy, processed carbs

Bagels

Cakes and other baked goods

Cereal (especially high-sugar cereal)

Cookies

Crackers and chips

Muffins

White bread, rolls, etc.

Fried anything!
French fries

Fried chicken

Fried onion rings

Other highly processed foods
Deli meats—from salami to bologna, maple turkey,
or ham

Prepared foods, including some "diet" meals—again,
look at the contents, and if they list preservatives
and high amounts of sodium, such foods can
backfire on your system!

Sweets
Brownies

Candy

Sauces
Bottled salad dressing

Creamy sauces

Ketchup

Mayonnaise

Drinks
Beer

Energy drinks

Fruit juice

Liquor

Soda or pop

Sweetened coffee and tea drinks

Wine

Miscellaneous culprits

Frozen dinner entrées (especially those high in sodium)

Protein or energy bars

What do these foods have in common? They tend to be

— high in sugar (this includes white, starchy carbs that turn to sugar and act like sugar when the body tries to break them down)
— high in hydrogenated fat
— high in sodium, which acts as an appetite stimulant
— high in chemicals and other preservatives that interfere with digestion and metabolism

Perhaps one or more of these common culprits appear more than once a day in your diet. Perhaps your hidden food isn't on this list, but you know in your heart that it is woven into your snacks and meals in a subtle but regular way.

Again, Step 2 asks you to remove the one, two, or three foods that you think you cannot live without. Maybe you need to cut them one at a time. That's fine.

Your Journal: Naming Your Hidden Foods

✼ Simply acknowledging a hidden food can feel very frightening. Your mind and body are so attached to hidden foods that just naming them, and writing them down in your journal, may be enormously difficult because this action is your first step to removing them from your life. As I said earlier, you may not be giving up these foods forever, but if any food is that powerful an interrupter to your body and your brain, then you need to think of its removal as at least semipermanent. For the next four weeks at minimum, you are going to stay away from these foods.

Think about this. Write about how you feel and all the thoughts and emotions that come up for you as you contemplate removing your hidden food or foods from your daily life.

Once you cut that food out of your diet and start to lose weight, you may begin looking at a deeper part of yourself, the part of you that has been hiding—from yourself and the world.

Very few of us can hide the fact that we're overweight, so what's so scary about losing that weight? Often, it's not the fat we're hiding. But we are hiding something. And it's not easy being honest with yourself about what that is. The truth often has the power of clarity, but it also can make us very uncomfortable. My advice? Give yourself permission to *feel whatever you feel* as you lose weight: sad, relieved, ashamed. Maybe you feel angry, frustrated, discouraged, helpless, or hopeless. *Just keep going.* Step by step. First step 1, then step 2. You will work through any obstacle in your way. Trust yourself. You can do it.

First: Take Action

Now that you have identified your hidden food, stop eating it for one week. That's it. You are going to get to four weeks. But for now, just embrace one week. You can cut out anything for one week, right?

As I described earlier, you may feel ready to eliminate more than one trigger food at a time and go cold turkey. That's fine, but it is quite a shock to the system. By all means, however, if you have the guts and the fortitude, then go for it!

But most of you, I am guessing, will feel more comfortable starting slowly and building up your confidence gradually as you ease the hidden foods out of your body one by one, week by week.

If you've identified cheese, for example, then it's cheese you need to stop eating.

If you've identified ice cream, don't even think about having a spoonful.

If you've identified white breads, rolls, bagels, muffins, or crackers—then it's time to remove these starchy carbs from your diet.

Begin with one week. Set this as one of your near goals. Keep a record (in your journal) of what you eat for each meal and snack. Write down how you are feeling—even if these are all negative emotions! For one week, you can do it! Because at the end of this week, you will feel so much better!

Adjusting to the New You!

At a basic body level, removing your hidden food is like breaking a physical addiction. Can regular food be addictive? Chemically it can be. The underlying components of unhealthy sugar, fat, and starch can hijack and change the way we taste flavors, whether we feel full, and how we feel after we eat in general. If your system has been used to having a certain food or feeling a certain way for a long time, when those tastes and feelings are taken away, it's common to feel some sort of withdrawal. This is especially true of sugar, sodium, gluten, and manufactured fats.

The good news is that the withdrawal doesn't last forever *and it doesn't affect whether you lose weight.* The time it takes for our body's natural chemistry to reset varies from person to person. For some it may take a year, for others two years, and still others even longer. *This does not mean you will stop losing weight* but it does mean that you will remain sensitive to your hidden food. The fastest way to reset your body is to completely avoid your hidden food, but if that's not possible, the idea is to limit it.

In the meantime, *do you have the power to manage the discomfort* you are feeling? You need to keep in mind that your physical, emotional, and mental discomfort is real and natural. Like any withdrawal, the mild distress you feel is an indication of the change and transformation you are going through. Recognize that your body speaks to you all day long. When you feel uncomfortable, take a minute to let that register as a sign from your body. It is working hard to cleanse itself and needs time to do it, but that is not a deal breaker for you. This discomfort is short-lived and on the other side is a feeling so wonderful you will never go back to eating garbage again. Be patient, kind, and gentle—especially with yourself. Treat yourself to a hot bath doused with Epsom salts to enhance toxin release, or allow yourself an extra sleep-in. Download some movies you've been waiting to see. Think of what you do when you're coming down with a cold— try that.

And in a way, isn't *physically feeling* this change happening kind of *exciting*?

You can also soften any feelings of discomfort by spending some extra time thinking about how you can take care of yourself in other, more permanent ways. If food has always been your companion and reward, then it's up to you to find other sources of comfort:

- Buy yourself a new pillow
- Treat yourself to a spa day—whether that's getting your nails done or going to a resort
- Take a trip or a long-awaited day off from work in which you drive to a place of natural beauty—a lake, river, the ocean, or a national or state park
- Visit a museum or art gallery
- Reach out to old friends—set regular phone dates
- Connect with the Start Here community online

- Go for a walk or visit a beautiful formal garden
- Give yourself permission for one day not to be hard on yourself

In other words, reward yourself, and remind yourself that you are trying to reset your body, mind, and spirit, and that process takes time and a *gentle approach*.

If You Are Having Trouble Identifying Your Hidden Foods

Still not sure what your culprit could be? My guess is that, as you keep reading, you will likely figure it out. Alternatively, you can work with the following list of common food culprits to help you determine the food or foods that you might be dependent upon. As a shortcut, remove the following foods from your everyday diet. Does that mean you can *never* have these foods ever again? Of course not, but the goal is to remove at least one of these for one to two weeks and see how you feel. This won't be easy, but think of it as an experiment: you are testing how your body feels without one of these foods. If you are reactive to one of these foods, then without it you will feel energetic; you will think more clearly and sleep better at night. Your digestion will improve.

If you remove one of these foods and don't notice a big difference in how you feel after one to two weeks, then it is probably not your trigger food. So go on to the next possibility, and remove that food for one to two weeks.

My hunch is that your hidden foods fall into one of these categories:

- Sugar—Desserts are an obvious target, but did you know that many sauces (such as barbecue sauce and ketchup) and bottled salad dressings (including ranch, thousand island, blue cheese, and even some Italian-style dressings) are high in sugar? Yes, even salty and savory foods have hidden sugar. For example, one tablespoon of ranch dressing could have as many as two or three grams of sugar, and "lite" versions have even more. Many processed meats like hot dogs and deli meats contain shocking amounts of sugar, too.

- White flour products—Take a look at your wheat bread, cookies, bagels, breakfast pastry, waffles, pancakes, and muffins. Also, if the ingredients don't list "whole wheat" first, you may be eating bread made from a combination of white flour and some wheat flour, plus wheat-colored additives. Some of this bread may also secretly include our first culprit—sugar. In general, many white flour products behave like sugar in your body. It is best to avoid them.

- Hydrogenated fats—Foods containing hydrogenated fats don't taste any better than those with non-hydrogenated fats, yet they are harder for our bodies to properly digest, and therefore cause a chain of events that keep us fat and contribute to disease. And like sugar in many processed foods, hydrogenated fats are "hidden" on ingredient lists where we don't think to look for them! Such foods include most of the manufactured snacks, chips, pretzels, cheese-flavored puffs, popcorn, tortilla chips, and other so-called junk foods, as well as margarine, vegetable shortening, nondairy dessert toppings, and donuts!

- Packaged foods or premade meals—Any food that is packaged is processed, and processed foods contain chemicals and sodium—which slow down your metabolism and contribute to the body's toxic load. More important, processed foods contain few nutrients, so you are robbing yourself of important ingredients that would otherwise keep you healthy. Since the body has not been satiated nutritionally it will keep asking for food. This is how it is possible for some people to eat entire family-size bags of chips. The body pays, however, in weight gain and disease.

These four offenders are often the ultimate source of weight gain because they dominate your metabolism, take over your appetite control system, and bury your natural ability to feel hungry and full.

With one, two, three, or all four of these culprits removed, you will begin to empty your body of anti-foods (see below!) and you will soon shed the unwanted weight that has been making you suffer.

As you take these all-important steps toward health and weight loss, it is important to be critical of what goes into your mouth. Success can come only if you begin to question the nutritional value of food and place that nutrition high on your priority list. Nutrient-dense foods may take more time to prepare, but that effort is worth it. Manufactured foods are not really foods at all; they are packaged anti-foods that have only one goal in mind—to get your money out of your pocket. Compare such products to the apple. All it wants to do is nourish you. Manufactured foods contain a host of chemicals and toxins that flood the body with non-nutrients, poisons, and ingredients taken out of context that contribute nothing to health or weight management. The end result is often obesity and disease. We must learn to question all foods before consuming them. The bottom line is you. Nutrient-dense, properly prepared, well-sourced whole foods make you healthy and lean.

Anti-foods = Anti-health

✳ Hydrogenated fats are a man-made fat with no purpose in the human diet. They insert themselves into the cell membrane, making it less flexible. The more rigid the cell, the less it is able to function properly, eroding your health. There is *no* place for these engineered fats in your Start Here program.

Excess sodium contributes to hypertension. Many manufactured foods contain much more than the recommended daily allowance of 2,300 milligrams. Steer clear of table salt and reach instead for natural, unrefined sea salt, which contains ninety-two valuable trace elements and minerals necessary for health.

Refined sugar is probably the biggest and most dangerous contributor to overweight and disease in the world. No other "food" has caused so much damage. It is highly addicting, contributes nothing to health, and actually robs the body of valuable stores of nutrients in its effort to process the white stuff. Avoid it at all costs.

GENTLE SHORTCUT: Dietproof Your Environment

One way to truly take care of yourself is to make your eating environment safe: that means tossing out any lingering hidden foods from your cupboards, refrigerator, freezer—or under your bed. You can never be too careful or take too many precautions when you are trying to remove your food triggers! Does that mean you'll never eat your hidden food? Of course not. The idea is simply to prevent yourself from unconsciously grabbing it in a moment of stress.

Here are some other tips to dietproof your environment:

- Clean out cupboards yourself.
- Avoid fast-food restaurants; take a new route from work to home or school if they are a temptation.
- Give yourself empowering visual cues, such as sticky notes on the refrigerator or the mirror in your bathroom or bedroom.
- Create a gentle, calm atmosphere in your home conducive to the tranquillity you are building on your inside.

Easy Guide to Food Groups

For our brains and bodies to function, we need to eat foods from the three main food groups—carbohydrates, protein, and fat. It's key to eat the right balance of these foods. I've noted those foods that you should *include, but enjoy in moderation* and those you should *limit*:

ENJOY IN MODERATION

- Protein that is low in negative fats—this includes lean well-sourced grass-fed meats, poultry, seafood, and fermented tofu (tempeh).
- Complex carbohydrates high in fiber—eat whole grains, fruits, and vegetables, with an emphasis on leafy greens.
- Legumes, such as beans and lentils—a mix of complex carbs and protein, these are also high in fiber. They pack a nutrient-rich punch without the fat of meat. Presoak for optimal nutrient value.
- Fats with the proper balance of omega-3, -6, and -9 fatty acids and no trans fats—these include olive oil, coconut oil, fish oil, and nuts and seeds and their oils.

LIMIT

- Simple carbohydrates—these carbohydrates contain high starch and/or sugar and are low in fiber. Found in breads, pastas, rice, potatoes, and sweets.
- Dairy—full fat dairy products, including milk, cheese, and yogurt, are an excellent source of protein; plain varieties are best rather than those loaded with sugar. Cheese should be limited.

In general, make sure all meals contain a balance of protein, healthy fat, and complex carbohydrates (again, these carbs need to be high in fiber). The fiber that is natural to fruits, vegetables, and whole grains is non-soluble and not only slows down the absorption rate of food, thus moderating the release of glucose into the blood, but also fills you up. But like any food, no matter how nutritious, fruit must be enjoyed in moderation as stated above. Fruits and vegetables cleanse the body of toxins, keep our metabolism working properly, and move the food along with ease. As most nutritionists will tell you, fiber is one of the simplest ways to ensure that your body stays clean and light. It may help you to remember the most healthy proportions of macronutrients:

30% fat

30% protein

40% carbohydrate: 20% leafy greens, 20% whole grains
     and fruit

As you get familiar with these categories, you will find it easier to make healthy food choices. Things get less straightforward and you are more likely to be deceived, however, when you turn to processed or packaged foods, which I prefer to call anti-foods.

The biggest reason behind the national obesity and diabetes crisis is our overconsumption of processed foods and our ignorance regarding proper nutrition, including fats. Engineered anti-foods are no longer strictly made up of ingredients from the food groups listed above, but have added agents that literally change their nature. To increase their shelf life and add flavor, processed foods are prepared with additives, including trans fats, sodium, excess refined and artificial sugars, and other harmful ingredients, all of which contribute to weight gain and disease. The bottom line? Our bodies are not meant to metabolize the ingredients added to manufactured foods that keep them "fresh" on the grocery store shelf, the freezer, or the cupboard. Try to eat fresh foods as much as you possibly can. And if you have to eat at a fast-food chain or from a package, make your choices wisely. Some fast food is relatively clean and healthy—instead of fried, go for grilled; skip the fries; and try to include a salad for fiber. Even though packaged foods can be overly processed, including sodium and all sorts of other additives, some brands are organic and/or healthy. The key is to look at the label of any packaged or frozen food and make sure the sodium count is below 500 mg, no MSG (monosodium glutamate) is included, and few, if any, artificial colors, sweeteners, or chemicals are listed. Also look at that label carefully to see how many words you can actually read. If there are none, don't eat that anti-food.

Portion Sizes

My guidelines for portion sizes are basic. Once you get used to these general serving sizes and you stick to eating healthy foods, you really don't have to worry about calories—you will automatically stay within the range for weight loss and/or maintenance. Most people find it easier to think of their foods in portion sizes, but the only foods you need to limit are protein, fats, and low-fiber carbohydrates. But you decide which strategy works for you. Some people like the portion guidelines; others prefer to restrict just the protein and fat and starchy carbs, eating as many vegetables and fruits as they like.

I am not the type to measure, weigh, or overthink my portion sizes. Instead, I eyeball amounts and then simply see how I feel. If I'm still hungry, I'll eat more; if I feel full, I'll stop eating. I let my body tell me what it needs. The following guidelines are based on healthy portion sizes that provide enough food to keep you satisfied. And if you wish to lose only a few pounds, these amounts will help you trim calories and reinforce the impact of your workouts so that you lose weight safely.

Here are some basic rules of thumb to follow each day:

Protein—fish, chicken, meat, legumes: Limit your protein intake to one piece of meat about the size of the palm of your hand.

Complex carbohydrates—fruit, vegetables, and whole grains: The portion size for whole grains should be two palmfuls; however, you can eat veggies to your heart's content. Because they are so loaded with fiber and vitamins, and act as a natural detox for your body, you can't eat too much—your body will utilize every ounce! Fruits should be eaten in moderation and not in unlimited quantities since they are still sugars, albeit natural.

Simple carbohydrates—bread, pasta, potatoes, couscous, rice: Keep your portions of grains to one fist if it's an accompaniment or two fists if it's the main dish (for example, rice topped with stir-fried veggies).

Unsaturated fats: Limit yourself to one to two tablespoons of natural nut butter or olive oil (for example, in a salad dressing).

Dairy: Milk, yogurt, and cheese are excellent sources of protein and calcium, but you do have to make good choices here and plain is always best. Also, much dairy is tainted with hormones and additives. Try to choose organic brands if you can and limit your portions to one cup.

Beverages

Whether your goal is to improve your fitness, lose pounds or inches, or both, it's important to keep well hydrated. However, you need to be conscious of and choosy about what you drink. Plain water is really the best, especially if you put a pinch of sea salt and a squeeze of lemon or lime in your glass. I DON'T DRINK SODA AND NEVER HAVE. I avoid all artificial sweeteners. None of them are good for anyone. Water is always best!

Fat Confusion

✒ Certain fats are required for optimal health and function. We need to get over our fear of fats and replace it with respect—as long as the fats you choose are healthful. Our brains need certain fats to function properly and, since our bodies don't produce these essential fatty acids, we must get them from other sources, such as fish oil, flaxseed, and coconut and olive oils. Better to choose high-quality fats—including some saturated fat, the preferred food for the heart and the brain—than to stuff ourselves with toxic and often rancid fats. The body cannot do without proper fats. Without them you have no metabolism, no immune system, no hormones, no "color," and no zest for life. It is important to make better choices about the fat we eat. I love fats from organic eggs, organic unsalted butter, nuts and seeds, and avocados—even dark leafy greens contain some omega-3 fats.

Reenvision Your Meals

As you get used to living without your hidden food, what will your meals look like? In the chapters that follow I provide suggestions for what might appear on your plate during your first week on the Start Here program, including recipes and shortcuts you'll love. But for now, let's have a little fun talking about all the foods *you will soon enjoy*.

Let's try this exercise together:

1. Take a blank sheet of paper, create a new document and folder on your laptop, or set up a new memo page on your phone.

2. Write down each food that typically makes up your breakfast.

3. Now compare that list with the suggestions below.

- **Healthy grains**
- **Lean proteins**
- **Fruits and vegetables for morning**

Tosca's Start Here Plate—What Your Daily Meals Should Look Like

Replating your food is a lot like TLC's hit show, *What Not to Wear.* In the show people learn to rethink what they wear by examining how their current dress style contributes—or doesn't—to their look. For your diet, the same can be accomplished by replating, where you take a hard look at what currently lands on your plate and "edit" it to nudge you in the direction of health and weight loss, and a better lifestyle overall. Like clothing, food contributes to how you look and feel. Some clothes look amazing on you and some do not. Food also can make you look amazing—or not. You know this is true because as you sit and read this you are feeling a desire to change something about your appearance. This is exactly where I began thirteen years ago. A simple tool like replating is a powerful way to see your food and portions differently.

On the Start Here plate, your first meal of the day can be loaded with the following foods. Many of the foods suggested here may already be your favorites, and you'll find many easy recipes at the back of this book.

Gorgeous Grains

Multigrain waffles with raspberries, protein pancakes, gluten-free raisin cinnamon scones, oatmeal with cranberries

Proteins That Please the Palate

Poached egg over asparagus, leftover bean chili, picante frittata

Fruits and Vegetables That Wake You Up and Fill You Up

Broiled grapefruit, salad with leftover grilled chicken for breakfast, a breakfast sausage sandwich!

These foods (and many more!) are delicious, easy on your system, and immediately set you up to feel satisfied, balanced, and grounded throughout the day. The careful but simple mix of grains, protein, and fruit or veggies ensures that you won't trigger your cravings for your hidden food. Even healthy fats are included to keep your hormonal and metabolic functions in high gear. The brain loves them, too.

If you start the day with a breakfast that contains one of your hidden foods, it becomes almost impossible to reset your body for the rest of the day. Those dangerous anti-foods zap your body's energy by giving you low nutrition when your body needs it most. Did you know we all wake up with low blood sugar and dehydrated? After a night's sleep, your body needs to have a rich blend of protein, complex carbs, and good fat to wake it up and start your day clearly.

Anti-foods break your body down, destroying your health and robbing you of the physique you want. Think of them in the same way as fuel for your car. Cheap gas makes your engine sputter and die. High quality makes your engine run like a race car. If you replate your breakfast and begin each day with one or two of these personal favorites, then you set yourself up for success! Breakfast also sets the tone for your day; a bad or good meal will make you feel bad or good. I opt for feeling my best whenever possible, so my breakfast looks like I mean business when it comes to nutrition. No donuts or pastries ever appear on my plate. Give me seeds, grains, protein, and healthy fat and I am ready to take on my day!

Replating Your Meals

Replating should not entail a lot of time or hassle. By having your new favorite breakfast foods on hand, you can save yourself a slipup. So next time you're at the grocery store, put these must-have items in your basket:

- Oatmeal
- Ezekiel bread (in the frozen food aisle)
- Raw almonds or almond butter
- Raw walnuts or walnut butter
- Raw pumpkin seeds
- Organic eggs
- Plain Greek yogurt
- Berries and apples

What you are doing is rethinking your meals. Is breakfast always pastry and donuts? Try salad greens with poached eggs. Or dust your morning salad with hemp hearts, fat ripe tomatoes, and a dollop of scrambled eggs.

Lunch will begin to look like this:

Green salad with grilled chicken
Quinoa Black Bean Burger with a side of fruit salad
Greek salad
Tuna with a squeeze of lemon and a side of tomato salad

Dinner will look like this:

Peanut Noodles with Chicken and Vegetables
Lemon and Herb Crusted Cod with Jojo Potatoes and
a side of steamed broccoli

One-Skillet Sweet and Sour Chicken with brown rice
   and steamed broccoli

And did I mention water? You will be drinking lots and lots of water! Water with lemon, water with orange, water with bubbles or without!

How Are You Doing?

Removing your hidden foods (step 2) is an amazing, empowering step toward a healthy new life. It's simple but not necessarily easy. Remember to use all your support tools to keep steady and focused on your near goals—what you want to accomplish in week 1. Then as you move into week 2, stop and reflect. Turn to your journal and record your thoughts and feelings. Are you still feeling anxious? Do you feel a bit more clearheaded, confident maybe? If you are indeed feeling stronger, then you are probably ready to tackle step 3 and begin to move a little. If, however, you feel you need more time just on step 2, that's absolutely fine. You can stay at week 1 as long as necessary, until you feel that inner trust begin to rise through you. That's the signal that you've made progress, that in this process called life, you are heading in the right direction!

As one client, Mary Ann, shared with me, "All I could do was take out my one hidden food—it was sugared cereal, which I used to eat day and night. I was so addicted, I couldn't ever imagine my life without it. I think I kept Kellogg's in business! In the end it took me four weeks of not eating cereal to finally have the guts to go on to step 2, but the wait was worth it. By that time, I had already lost ten pounds and felt so much more ready to start moving!"

Being ready is all up to you!

5

Step 3: Move a Little

By simply removing your hidden food from your diet *you will lose weight*. Why is that? Most people don't believe it, but more than half of all weight loss success is due to a change in what you eat, period. By simply cutting out the food culprits in your life, you will lose weight with less effort than you ever have before.

And again, some people stick with that step for weeks before incorporating step 3. Other people do the steps together. Jake said that he wanted to "go for it" by taking out his hidden foods (fried seafood, French fries, chicken fingers) and then hiring a personal trainer. In less than three months, he had lost thirty-two pounds and felt "ripped." Of course, not everyone can afford a trainer, and many people need to start moving in a more modest way before engaging in more strenuous physical activities, including sports. Which is why step 3 includes the word *little*!

What's involved in the next step?

In step 3, I am asking you to move . . . *a little*. I'm not asking you to join a gym, start jogging, or invest in a treadmill. Those exercise options are out there—yes. But all you need to do in the Start Here program is go from *not* moving to moving *a little*. That's it.

In this chapter you will find three lists to choose from: the first is a list of twenty-five everyday activities; the second, twenty-five basic, easy movements; and the third, twenty-five sport-like activities to get your heart pumping and your muscles aching!

You naturally encounter most of these familiar movements in your daily life. You don't have to buy any equipment, and you don't have to commit to an hour-long program. Even better, you don't have to feel intimidated by gym junkies.

All you have to do is familiarize yourself with the list of activities and begin to move—just a little—each day. I work with women and men all around the country and the world, all busy and distracted, yet every one of these clients has been able to fit a handful of these activities into their regular schedules. One of the best bodies I ever saw belonged to a woman from Australia who walked everywhere, up hill and down, and that effort alone paired with proper eating got her ripped. For example, you could:

> Walk up the stairs instead of riding an elevator
> Iron for fifteen minutes
> Take an extra lap around the office
> Sweep the floor or vacuum

Integrating these movements into your day and week may take some extra thought in the beginning as you familiarize yourself with your options, but soon enough you will be doing these activities regularly. For now, you don't even need to think about time or duration. Simply move. I love to vacuum. During stressful times I still pull out the vacuum cleaner and get nice and sweaty cleaning my house. The bonus is the house sparkles!

Now let's get started!

First Things First: Health Checkup

✎ Depending on your current activity level, you should check in with your doctor, physical therapist, or nurse practitioner before starting step 3 of your Start Here plan.

It's always a good idea to know where you stand in terms of important health measurements; with that in mind, ask your physician to give you a routine physical to gather the following information:

> Blood pressure
> Cholesterol
>> *HDL (good cholesterol)*
>> *LDL (bad cholesterol)*
> Blood sugar
> Weight
> BMI (body mass index) (see page 227 for more information
>> about how to interpret your BMI)
> Waist-to-hip ratio

It's also important to review your medications so your doctor can share any information related to side effects. None of what you do in the Start Here plan is remotely life-threatening; in fact your health and life will improve, but it is important to be sure you have no unexpected risk factors. For more specific information regarding healthy numbers for these tests, refer to the Resources section at the back of the book.

25 Ways to Move a Little

The following exercises are really just little movements you can incorporate into your day. They are suggestions, not guidelines; you might think of lots of other little movements that fit into your daily life just from reading these. Peruse the list and think about those movements that work in your lifestyle. Ask yourself if they seem realistic, given how and where you spend the majority of your day. If you work in an office, for example, putting away the laundry piece by piece is probably not realistic. If you work from home or are a homemaker, then putting away laundry makes more sense than, say, walking the stairs in your office building.

25 Gentle Movements

- Put laundry away piece by piece.
- Wash the dishes.
- Wash down the refrigerator inside and out.
- Go up and down the stairs, slowly at first.
- Plant flowers or vegetables or pick weeds in the garden.
- Take a special trip to the mailbox.
- Vacuum while holding in your stomach.
- Walk your block or around your office building during your coffee break.
- Park your car far from the entrance to the grocery store.
- Walk when you would otherwise take a taxi.
- Dust tops of window frames, fans, and other high places.
- Wipe down the walls in two rooms of your house or apartment.
- Wash the windows in one room of your house or apartment.
- Sweep the floors.
- Push a stroller.
- Vacuum the car.

- Move the furniture and vacuum behind it.
- Paint a piece of furniture.
- Sit on the edge of the sofa and lift one leg, straightening your knee, while watching your favorite TV show, alternating legs.
- Sit on the edge of the bed and raise your arms up and down in continuous motion as you think about your meal choices for the day.
- Clean out the tub.
- Go apple picking or take a walk to a nearby park or nature preserve.
- Walk the mall or business district by your home.
- While sitting at your desk or the kitchen table, lift your feet up and down as if you were marching in place.

Do you see a pattern? These movements are designed for people who already have a full plate of chores, so each of these movements—or any you might add—are designed to help you finish work that you have to do anyway.

But be intentional when you engage in these activities. Be purposeful. For example, when putting away the laundry, stand firmly on your feet and hold in your belly. When you pay attention to your feet and push into them as you contract your abdominal muscles, you activate your core and strengthen your overall posture.

Many people who have been sedentary and are not used to physical exertion lose a sense of balance and often feel unsteady on their feet. When you begin moving in simple ways but with an awareness of how you are moving, you will gradually improve your balance and strength.

Begin by devoting fifteen to twenty minutes to one or two movements three to five days a week. As I indicated in the previous chapter, don't get too far ahead of yourself. Instead, take it week by week, especially in the first three weeks of your Start Here journey. Try activities *one at a time* and *limit your movement* to fifteen to twenty minutes until you feel comfortable with the movement. Then consider extending your activity time to thirty to forty minutes, or simply adding a second movement until you find yourself active for thirty to forty minutes. Look at the list below and consider your options.

So for now, here's what to do:

1. Choose one, two, or three activities from the list above.
2. In your calendar or journal, mark five to seven 15-minute periods to incorporate movement during the day over the course of a week.
3. If you feel ready, combine movements in different ways:

   Two 15-minute sessions in the morning
   One 30-minute session in the morning
   Three 15-minute sessions—one in the morning, two in the afternoon
   One 60-minute session

You get the idea! As you will see in chapter 8, where I have designed a four-week program, you can create your own combinations at whatever time of day best works for you. And what best works for you is the time that you are most likely to move a little!

Renee was a tennis player when she was young, but gave it up after college. Since then, she's packed on the pounds—twenty-five to be exact. She was feeling grumpy and groggy all the time, and complained of frequent headaches. After removing her hidden food (she lived on pasta—especially with thick, creamy, cheesy sauces!), she began by doing simple tasks around her house. She was handy, so she decided to put together a bookshelf. This project led to another: she decided to clean out her basement!

Within a month of giving herself these everyday chores, she actually felt inclined to pick up her tennis racquet again. But she had to take it easy. Her legs were weak and unsteady, and her knees were achy because the muscles of her thighs had atrophied.

Yet she persevered. Six months later, she was playing tennis on a weekly basis—not only getting into better shape but enjoying herself immensely.

Start small. Keep your near goals in mind and try not to get ahead of yourself. If you haven't been moving and your body is weak from disuse, then it will take some time to feel strong enough to try activities that require a bit more exertion.

Once you are comfortable adding these movements to your life, you will feel up for a challenge and ready to commit to movement that is slightly more demanding. In addition to the movement that your body will enjoy, can you imagine how clean your home will be?

Fitting Movement into Your Schedule

Like me, many of you may have lives that seem to get increasingly busy, with longer work days and crazier schedules, so it may seem unreasonable to include one more thing! But try and move away from that line of thinking and give yourself a new direction: imagine that by including just a small amount of physical activity, you are actually doing something that will increase your overall energy level.

There are many ways to fit movement into your life. Instead of plopping yourself in front of the TV to eat your lunch, eat at the kitchen table and then take a five- to ten-minute walk. My guess is that if this becomes a habit, your walk will soon extend to fifteen or twenty minutes! We all know about parking our cars farther away from the grocery store or office building. How about parking our bodies farther from our destinations by getting off the bus or train a stop sooner? Or walking three or four blocks past your destination and back? You will find that once you get moving, you will feel more inclined to move. You will actually miss those days when you don't have that activity!

You also want to think ahead: When are you most likely to fit in your physical activity? If you are a morning person, then it's probably best to plan on moving a little in the first half of the day. If you are slow to rise and tend to be a night owl, then late afternoon or early evening movement sessions are likely best for you. I have to look at my weekly schedule and fit in the days I will train along with my other responsibilities; otherwise I may be inclined to skip my movement date.

Personally, I like to work out first thing in the morning. I eat a quick, simple breakfast of a banana and ½ cup plain yogurt—enough to get my blood sugar in balance—and then I exercise for twenty to forty minutes. That way, once my day becomes hectic—and it always does—I know I have already given my body that special time.

But moving in the early morning is not for everyone—it really depends on what works for *you*, and what is most realistic for *you*.

Moving is important for overall health, but it also has the added benefit of supporting the removal of your hidden foods. Remember: you *will* lose weight *simply by cutting out your hidden foods*. So if you like what you see in the mirror, *add* a little movement to your routine in order to *step up your pace of weight loss*. The following list of easy movements will take your activity up a notch.

Remember, muscle tone and strength are built over time. The power of repetition is persuasive: it primes your muscles to respond to the movements, strengthening and toning them. Doing something like lifting for twenty minutes or leg raises for twenty minutes will help strengthen muscles, whereas doing different movements that are more cardio based (such as walking) might help you burn more calories but not necessarily pinpoint a particular area. As you combine different activities—some of them stretching, some of them strengthening, some of them increasing your cardio capacity—think of them as a gentle circuit training so that you get into the habit of engaging your entire body.

25 Easy Movements to Step Up Your Weight Loss

Consider the following moderate movements, which are longer in duration than those in the first list and a bit more complex, to step up your weight loss. As you try some of these movements, I recommend extending the duration for at least twenty to thirty minutes instead of the fifteen to twenty suggested above.

- Walk around the block, bending your arms at the elbows and gently swinging them forward and back as you walk.
- Vacuum the entire house while holding in your stomach muscles for thirty seconds at first, and then—if you can—for sixty seconds at a time.
- Wash the windows of your entire house or those inside your apartment, concentrating on using your biceps.
- Walk to the grocery store, the post office, or a friend's house for a sustained twenty to thirty minutes.
- Push a stroller around the park, pulling in your tummy and exerting your arms with intention.
- Take a long walk in a park or wooded area, stopping every fifteen minutes to do knee lifts in place for five minutes.
- Walk on a treadmill, keeping your arms at your sides but moving them back and forth as you walk.
- Hold a can of food in each hand and do arm lifts from a standing position while listening to the radio or watching TV. Make sure you keep your shoulders down when you lift your arms overhead.
- Sit on the edge of a sofa or bed and lean down from side to side

while watching your favorite TV show; this torso twist helps stretch out your abdomen and back muscles.

- Clean out the garage or storage unit. When lifting or moving heavy objects, make sure you pull in from your stomach and don't overuse your back.
- Walk up and down the stairs two times, building up to five times.
- From the bottom step, step backward down and up, down and up; you should feel this in the back of your thighs (your hamstrings) and in your butt (your glutes).
- While sitting at your desk, in your car, or on the subway, sit up straight and pull in your stomach muscles, first for thirty seconds at a time, then for sixty seconds at a time, for a period of fifteen minutes.
- Walk your dog at a fast pace around the block; remember to breathe as you increase the duration from fifteen to twenty minutes and then twenty to thirty minutes.
- Lie on your bed and do scissor kicks while watching TV. Remember: keep that tummy tight.
- Pack up boxes of clothes you no longer wear; carry them to the car or a taxi, and take them to a charity or resale shop.
- From a standing position, raise your knees one at a time while watching your kids or reading a book; after five minutes, try to touch your knee to one elbow and then alternate sides.
- From a standing position, touch your toes, then squeeze your butt muscles when you straighten up.
- Standing with your legs wide apart (about the width of a yoga mat), bend your knees as if you were sitting on a chair, sticking your butt out and keeping your back straight; gently move up and down. You will feel this squat in your thighs, the back of your legs, and your butt.
- Raise your arms overhead and circle them backward and then

forward while watching TV; these arm extensions open your shoulders, back, and the muscles across your chest.

- Raise your arms out to your sides and flex your fingers up and down.
- Lie on your back, tuck your legs into a loose fetal position, and stretch your knees to one side. Stay in this position for five to ten minutes; then alternate sides. These easy stretches are wonderful hip and back openers.
- Sit up straight in a chair and turn your head gently to the right, back to center, and then to the left while listening to music or an audio book. This easy movement unlocks your neck and helps maintain posture.
- Lie on your back and place your hands behind your head; cradle your head without straining your neck. Now do ten gentle crunches, pulling in your stomach muscles as you raise your upper body off the floor. Remember: don't lift from your neck!
- Lie on your back and tuck your chin toward your chest; this easy neck roll helps to keep your spine and neck soft and pliable.

These movements can be done by themselves for fifteen, twenty, or thirty minutes or combined for an even longer duration. The key is to decide to do *three or four activities (from either list) each week*, trying to do *at least one each day*.

The more you move, the more you will feel like moving. So if all you can do the first week is one 15-minute activity, don't sweat it.

By next week, you will feel different—you will feel better and more ready to increase the duration and the frequency of your movements. That's when you want to think about pairing different activities: fifteen minutes of one activity in the morning, then twenty minutes of another during lunch, then fifteen minutes after coming home from work. If you don't like splicing it up, then pair up activities in one or two segments, again thinking about when you are most likely to follow through.

Tom loved doing three 15-minute segments—stretches when he woke up at 6:30 A.M.; a walk around the office complex at lunchtime; and a fifteen-minute session on his StairMaster when he got home from work and before he enjoyed his dinner. There are really easy ways of fitting in these little movements throughout the day—and they will start adding up to a lot of movement. Then you can ease into a more intense type of activity, duration, and frequency.

You may find it helpful to create one place in your kitchen—maybe an erasable whiteboard—where you list the activities and easy movements that you want to incorporate for that week. That way you'll walk by your list every day. Each week, revise your list to keep activities fresh and fun. Or challenge yourself to go for a longer duration. You can also change the sequences. The more you change it up, the more you will motivate yourself.

Each one of us has our own goals for moving a little. What are yours? Here are some other inspiring goals that women and men have shared with me:

> Suzanne: "to change from an XXL to an XL"
> Mark: "to dance at my sister's wedding"
> Karen: "to really taste food again"
> Barbara: "to keep losing weight"
> Henry: "for my psoriasis to go away"
> Diane: "to get off my blood sugar medicine"

Your Journal: Reflect on Your Goals

✒ In your journal, reflect upon your near goals for fitness. *Why* do you want to move a little?

Write down, draw, or make a note on your phone of your near goals. Keep these ideas as simple and specific as possible.

What types of movement are you going to commit to this week?

Look at your schedule. Find four 15-minute slots.

Now step back for a minute, and imagine the benefits. Say your goal out loud. *Move a little.*

Going the Distance: Burn Baby Burn

As some of you may know from my previous books, one of the biggest transformations of my adult life happened to me after I turned forty. I had met my husband, Robert, who happened not only to be the publisher of *Oxygen,* the women's fitness magazine, but also a former body builder himself. He and I clicked in a lot of ways, but one important thing he did was help me frame one of my far goals: after living a fat and frumpy life, I aspired to reshape my physique and get on the cover of *Oxygen* magazine. Yes, I did it! But it wasn't easy, and it took time and a lot of willpower.

The activities on this next list have the potential to push your body into even better shape. Please don't try these right out of the box; first give yourself time to heal on the inside, remove your hidden food, and move a little. But when you are ready—and you will know when that is—you just might enjoy the extra challenge of these activities.

The Challenge List:
25 Activities to Move Your Muscles

- Circuit training
- Cycling
- Dancing (line)

- Golf
- Hiking
- Elliptical machine
- Kickboxing
- Mountain biking
- Pilates
- Power yoga (Ashtanga)
- Boot camp or muscle pump class
- Rock climbing
- Rowing
- Running/jogging
- Cross-country skiing
- Squash
- Spin class
- StairMaster
- Swimming
- Tai chi
- Tae Bo
- Tennis
- Triathlon
- Weight lifting
- Zumba
- Cross fit
- Endurance events

Calorie Burning Chart

Your weight loss and dietary results will no doubt be enhanced by your physical activities. As one woman I know put it, "Nothing motivates me to stay away from the pantry like realizing that a serving of chips and hummus (which I think of as healthy, since at least it's not sugary or fried!) is equal to the hour I just spent walking home from work."

Take a look at the following chart and consider the calories you can burn doing these everyday activities, as well as some exercises that are more rigorous.

Calorie Burning Guide

Activity	15 minutes	30 minutes	45 minutes	60 minutes
Walking (flat)	65	130	200	275
Walking (hills)	90	180	260	380
Weeding a garden	90	160	230	320
Bike riding	75	130	190	240
Childcare	76	155	320	400
Circuit training	178	355	533	711
Cycling	100	200	300	410
Dancing (line)	65	138	195	258
Golf	45	115	170	230
Aerobics (low impact)	135	270	400	540
Elliptical machine	125	400	425	575
Grocery shopping	76	155	320	400

Activity	15 minutes	30 minutes	45 minutes	60 minutes
Planting	89	178	267	356
Playing with kids	89	178	267	356
Raking lawn	89	178	267	356
Running/ jogging	180	360	540	730
StairMaster	155	310	460	618
Stretching	89	178	267	356
Sweeping	89	178	267	356
Swimming	130	250	380	510
Tai chi	89	178	267	356
Tennis	110	225	350	450
Vacuuming	89	178	267	356
Washing car	84	167	251	335
Yoga	70	120	185	240

Source: Harvard Medical School: http://www.health.harvard.edu/

Rewarding Yourself for Steps Well Taken

Many of us want to reward ourselves with "cheat meals" or "cheat days" that allow us to return to our hidden foods or skip a day or two of movement. Sure, you can do this on the Start Here program and still continue to lose weight (so long as you return to the program!). But consider this: the *real* reward is what happens when you lose weight and feel great—when your health returns *because* you've removed your hidden foods, moved a little, or both. What could be better? Once you feel this, other rewards (like cheat days) become less important. *After all, what could possibly taste as good as feeling lighter and healthier?* If you're looking for rewards outside of yourself, you are probably not motivated by your own goals. This can trigger bad habits. So make sure that your rewards align with your goals. Do you feel better? Then you're on the right track. What a great reward!

As you come out of hiding, taking your new place may feel wonderful, but also a bit overwhelming. You may feel uncomfortable because you're not used to putting yourself and your health—even how you look!—first. But remember this: true learning and lasting change in life tend to come out of our most difficult challenges, and for you to grow, the ground will sometimes feel a little shaky under your feet. But this is not going to stop you from getting to your best self ever.

And of course, no matter how carefully we plan our lives, or how cautiously we live—and how well we are doing in our program—we will always face some form of external adversity. Whether that challenge or stress comes from a job change or loss, a new addition to the family, financial worries or woes—you need to feel ready to address things other than your internal challenge. I'm not suggesting that you stay poised, expecting bad things to happen; rather, I'm saying don't waste your energy being surprised when difficult events occur. The true test of your vision of your new self is when life gets complicated. Instead of retreating to familiar, comforting habits, remind yourself that you are ready to take on or absorb this new challenge. So as you remove your hidden food, begin to move a little, and list your goals, keep reminders of the things and people you can call on to support you when you feel less strong—to help you stay on track with each part of the Start Here plan.

Ultimately, I encourage you to allow the *simplicity* of the Start Here plan to serve as a support system. It's just three things—certainly you can take one of these steps on most days? Use these three steps, as a backbone, a support system, and a best friend you can always rely on. Rely on them, believe in them, and trust in them. I did, and they helped me make all my dreams come true. And if you take these steps, too, they will lead you to the new life you have always dreamed of.

What Are the Benefits of Moving *a Little*?

Moving a little seems so simple. What can it possibly do for you?

We've all heard about the importance of exercising. But no one really tells us how *regular movement* has an impact on our shape and metabolism. When you begin doing these movements routinely for fifteen to twenty minutes a day, you will not only maximize the impact of removing your hidden food, you will also wake up your body and feel more in touch with yourself. You will feel lighter, look leaner, and have more energy. You will be more alert to how certain foods, including but not limited to your hidden foods, make you feel. You will become more trusting of yourself, more confident. This is what *taking your place* really means. You are taking charge of yourself, your health, and your life.

PART THREE

Renovating Day by Day

6

Start Here Essentials: Shopping, Preparing, and Other Kitchen Shortcuts

I love to shop, cook, and spend time in the kitchen—but I know not everyone shares this passion. So I've gathered what I call my "shortcuts" that will help you fret less and enjoy more!

In this chapter you will find not only a complete grocery list to match the meal plans and recipes that follow, but also practical tips on preparing, cooking, and storing foods. I also spend some time on shopping strategies—so you stay away from the danger zone of the grocery store or market and get accustomed to shopping in a more strategic way.

All of this information will soon lead to your very own shortcuts to a happy and healthy lifestyle!

Dietproof Reminder

✿ Remember how I asked you to dietproof your environment? I can't emphasize enough the power of this step to help you prepare for the biggest change in your life. Before we head to the grocery store and begin to prepare the nurturing foods that you are about to enjoy, let's go back into your kitchen: Have you removed the trigger foods lurking in your refrigerator, cupboards, and other hiding places? I encourage you to take one more walk-through and remove all the offending foods so that when you return from your first trip to the market, you will be ready to go and primed for success!

Tosca's Journal

I always tell the girls that life's never perfect. It takes work. It takes discipline. But it also takes laughter and kindness. Be kind, Tosca!

Before Heading to the Grocery Store

Plan ahead! Grocery stores can be perilous places! Why? Because not everything you see loaded onto shelves and into coolers and cases is food. Much of it is anti-food—things you put in your mouth that don't nurture or feed you in the most basic way possible. Lining many shelves in supermarkets are box after box of manufactured food, processed in a lab with, it seems, one end goal: to pull your hard-earned money out of your pocket without actually contributing to your health. These foods—boxed cereals, snack food, cakes and cookies, chips, pretzels, and soda—tend to be rich in calories and poor in nutrition—almost empty, in fact. So my first caveat when shopping: shop the perimeter of the store where the fresh foods are placed!

Second, don't go food shopping when you are hungry or tired. Hungry shoppers make less than stellar decisions—even the most disciplined of us will begin to fill the cart with impulse purchases that are typically our go-to comfort foods—ice cream, cheese, and other trigger foods. To truly plan in advance, have a healthy snack before heading to the store!

Third, you must go with a list in hand (or on your smartphone). What do you need for the week or a few days? Have you perused the grocery list (at the end of this chapter) or the meal plans (in chapter 7)? Even if you might change your mind, it's a good idea to sketch out a plan for two or three meals and your favorite snack foods so that your refrigerator, cupboard, and fruit bowl are plentiful. Again, you don't want to find yourself hungry after a long day, then desperately dialing for a pizza!

The grocery list on page 112 offers an abundant variety of produce, meats, healthy dairy options, the best sauces, and salad fixings. I expect some of these may be new to you. It will take some time to familiarize yourself with foods you are not in the habit of preparing or enjoying. But please know that everything on this list is easy to prepare—and delicious!

Whether you are shopping for yourself or your entire family, it's a good idea to think about the food you will need for the upcoming few days. It may seem a bit tedious to plan an entire week in advance, but charting four or five days ahead can help you stick with your Start Here plan, and it's probably good for your wallet, too—you will avoid impulse purchases at take-out joints or restaurants if you already have menus in mind. Ultimately this planning is both a time- and lifesaver. I credit most of my success with eating and maintaining a slim physique today to planning. Don't underestimate its importance.

If you've gone ahead and looked at the meal plans, you may have already chosen some meals for the next few days. Make a list of the items that you don't already have on hand. You may also enjoy perusing the grocery list below and coming up with inspired lunch or dinner options.

At the Grocery Store

Is it a maze? Is it a casino? Is it Disneyland? Grocery stores nowadays offer everything from food to tires to computers and clothing. No wonder we often feel overwhelmed. Never mind the prices! With your list in hand, however, you will be able to resist the temptation to purchase what you don't need.

Again, I always suggest that you shop the perimeter of the store first—this is where the fresh produce, meat counters, dairy, and frozen food aisles typically are arranged. These food categories make up the majority of your list—they represent the nutritious foods that should be the basis of your diet.

Once you fill your cart with these wholesome necessities, you can venture toward the inside where the processed and packaged foods can usually be found. Keep your list handy so that you can skip certain aisles (candy! soda! packaged snacks!) and simply head to the ones where you can find your healthy condiments, water choices, grains, and other staples.

Reading Labels

✒ Most foods today are marked with labels that offer a breakdown of their "Nutrition Facts." Understanding how to read these labels is enlightening and gives you power over your food choices. Such labels tell you about the main ingredients of any food item so you can more knowedgeably select what goes into your cart and your mouth.

A very good rule of thumb is if you cannot pronounce the name of an ingredient, it is probably bad for you and it does not occur in nature; in other words, it's a chemical (or chemical compound) being used by food manufacturers for taste or as a preservative.

The nutrition label also provides the amounts of carbohydrate (including sugar), fat, protein, and sodium. This is often where you can find the hidden sugar and sodium—the two big offenders.

Nutrition Facts Serving Size 1 ounce Servings in bag 4	
Amount Per Serving	
Calories 155 Calories from Fat 93	
	% Daily Value*
Total Fat 11g	16%
Saturated Fat 3g	15%
Trans Fat	
Cholesterol 0mg	0%
Sodium 148mg	6%
Total Carbohydrate 14g	5%
Dietary Fiber 1g	5%
Sugars 1g	
Protein 2g	
Vitamin A 0% Vitamin C 9%	
Calcium 1% Iron 3%	

*Percent Daily Values are based on a 2,000 calorie diet. Your daily values may be higher or lower depending on your calorie needs.

Shopping Organic

You probably guessed this already: I highly suggest that you buy as much organic produce, dairy, meat, and fish as possible. Why? Organic foods do not contain harmful chemicals from pesticides and preservatives; many of these chemicals have been linked to disease, including cancer. Selecting organic food supports small local farmers, who are paid a fairer price for their organic produce. Most organic produce and other foods are local—without chemicals to preserve them, they have a much shorter "shelf life." They are also often at their nutritional peak.

Although organic foods are becoming more readily available (even Walmart offers an array of organic foods!), they tend to be more expensive. So if you have to choose, consider this list (often called the Dirty Dozen by the Environmental Working Group). These foods, because of their porous nature and thin skins, absorb the greatest amount of pesticides and other toxins and are best eaten organic:

1. Apples
2. Bell peppers
3. Celery
4. Cherries
5. Grapes
6. Nectarines
7. Peaches
8. Pears
9. Potatoes
10. Raspberries
11. Spinach
12. Strawberries

The twelve fruits and vegetables that have thicker skin and are therefore less harmful if not organic are:

1. Asparagus
2. Avocados
3. Bananas
4. Broccoli

5. Cauliflower

6. Corn

7. Kiwis

8. Mangoes

9. Onions

10. Papayas

11. Pineapples

12. Sweet peas

A Basic Guide to Shopping for and Cooking with Natural Foods

↗ Cooking with and enjoying natural foods offers a wonderful advantage: delicious taste, bountiful nutrition, and simple preparation. Here are some basic guidelines for enjoying and cooking with natural foods:

- Include mostly seasonal, organic fruits and vegetables.
- Avoid foods with artificial ingredients, including flavorings, colors, preservatives, and sweeteners.
- Use whole grains and unbleached flours.
- Avoid any food products that contain hydrogenated fats.
- Cook with ingredients as close to their natural state as possible, with minimal processing.
- Buy poultry, fish, and beef raised without the use of growth stimulants and antibiotics.

Tosca's Journal

Just came home with a bag of parsnips! Wonder what I will do with them today! Parsnip soup? The girls will LOVE it . . . or maybe not!

Your Grocery List

Fruits *(preferably fresh)*

Apples

Bananas

Berries (blueberries, blackberries, strawberries)

Cherries

Kiwis

Lemons

Limes

Mandarin or navel oranges

Peaches

Pears

Pineapples

Vegetables

Asparagus

Bean sprouts

Cabbage

Carrots

Celery

Corn (fresh or frozen)

Cucumbers

Eggplants

Frozen peas

Grape tomatoes

Kale

Leeks

Lettuce (romaine, Bibb, or red or green leaf)

Mushrooms

Plum tomatoes

Red and green peppers

Red onions

Scallions

Shallots

Spinach

Sweet potatoes

Yellow onions

Zucchini

Herbs (fresh)

Basil

Chiles

Chives

Cilantro

Coriander

Flat-leaf parsley

Garlic

Gingerroot

Mint

Oregano

Rosemary

Raw Nuts and Seeds and Dried Fruits

Almonds

Cashews

Dried cranberries

Nut and seed butters

Peanuts

Pine nuts

Pumpkin or sunflower seeds

Raisins

Grains

Arborio rice

Brown rice (long-grain)

Bulgur

Flaxseed

Oat bran

Quinoa

Rice noodles

Rolled oats

Wheat germ

Dairy

Butter (Organic is best.)

Cottage cheese

Eggs (Free range are best.)

Milk

Parmesan cheese

Yogurt

Meat and Fish

Chicken breasts

Flounder or tilapia fillets

Lean ground beef or bison

Lean ground chicken

Lean ground turkey

Salmon fillets

Shrimp

Legumes

Black beans

Chickpeas

Edamame

Kidney beans

Lentils

Pinto beans

Breads

Ezekiel bread

Whole-wheat bread

Whole-wheat or corn tortillas

Spices

Allspice

Basil

Black pepper

Cayenne pepper

Chili powder

Cinnamon

Cloves, ground

Coriander

Cumin

Fennel seed

Garlic powder

Garlic salt

Nutmeg

Oregano

Paprika

Parsley

Red pepper flakes

Rosemary

Sea salt

Thyme

Stocks, Pastes & Oils

Chili paste

Coconut milk and oil

Eat-Clean Spray

Low-sodium chicken stock

Olive oil

Peanut oil

Toasted sesame oil

Tomato paste

Sweeteners

Honey

Maple syrup

Molasses

Vinegars

Apple Cider

Balsamic

Rice wine

Sauces

Hot sauce

Low-sodium soy sauce

Worcestershire sauce

Baking

Almond meal

Arrowroot flour

Baking soda

Cornstarch

Spelt or whole-wheat flour

Vanilla extract

Kitchen Equipment

Even if you don't aspire to become a chef, your enjoyment and preparation of food will improve tremendously if you invest in some high-quality—though not necessarily expensive—pots and pans and other utensils. You do not need a large number, but it's important to have a good selection:

A good set of knives for dicing, paring, and carving,
    plus serrated for slicing

Colander

Grater

Heavy-bottomed saucepan for grains

Kitchen tongs

Large slotted spoon

Measuring cups and spoons

Roasting pan

Sauté pan (6- and 9-inch for chicken, shrimp, etc.)

Set of wooden spoons in different sizes

Soup ladle

Spatulas

Steamer

Vegetable peeler

Wok

Cooking Prep Tips

I love to cook! I enjoy the creativity of the process, the delicate work with food and spices, and the results—whether eating on my own or sharing what I've prepared with my family. I do know, however, that not all of you share my passion nor do you have the time to fit this into your busy lives. Please know that the meals (in the next chapter) and the recipes (in chapter 10) are all *fast and easy* to prepare. That said, here are some general time-saving tips that will support you as you cook:

- Once you've chosen your meal or recipe, it's important to get out all the ingredients before you begin.
- Read the recipe the whole way through so you have a sense of its order, prep, and timing.
- Prepare your meats and vegetables on separate cutting boards.
- Slice, dice, and chop all meat or veggies before you begin to cook.

Storing and Cooking Your Natural Foods

The recipes and meal plans are easy to prepare. Keep in mind that though I love to cook, I am not a chef. I have an enormously busy schedule managing the many moving parts of my career, so my food has to work for me; I don't want to work for my food. Here are some suggestions I use myself to simplify food preparation and cooking. I have organized this practical advice by food group so that when any meal or recipe calls for a veggie, carb, meat, or fish, you will know exactly where to look for advice on cooking.

Grains

Rice and other grains are very simple to cook, and contrary to what many assume, they don't take a long time. All you need to figure out is how much water to match with the amount of grain you are preparing. If time permits, I add one step to the preparation of grains: I soak them the night before. So if I want Irish oats the next morning, I soak them overnight in a bowl of water. This helps release the nutrients stored in the grains, making them more readily available. Soaking also hastens cooking time.

The rule of thumb for cooking white rice is 2 cups water to 1 cup rice. For brown rice and other grains, use 1¾ cups water to 1 cup rice.

Typically, I prepare at least two or three days' worth of rice or grains, so that I can enjoy them with other meals or as leftovers. To extend the freshness of your cooked grains, simply refrigerate in an airtight container.

Grain (1 cup)	Liquid (cups)	Cooking Method*	Cooking Time**	Yield (cups)
Amaranth	3	Simmer	15 min.	2⅔
Barley, grits	⅔	Cereal	3 min. + 5 min. standing time	2
Barley, hulled	4	Simmer	1 hour 45 min.	2½
Barley, pearl	3	Simmer	45–55 min.	4
Barley, quick	2	Simmer	10–12 min.	3
Buckwheat, groats, unroasted	2	Cereal	15 min.	3½

Grain (1 cup)	Liquid (cups)	Cooking Method*	Cooking Time**	Yield (cups)
Buckwheat, groats, roasted	2	Cereal	15 min.	3
Corn, meal	4	Cereal	10 min.	3½
Corn, hominy, dried	5	Simmer	5–6 hours	3
Millet	3	Simmer	25–30 min. + 10 min. standing time	5
Oats, quick	2	Cereal or steep	1 min. + 3–5 min. standing time	2
Oats, old-fashioned	2	Cereal	5 min.	2
Oats, steel-cut	4	Cereal	20 min.	2
Quinoa	2	Simmer	15 min.	4
Rye, berries	3	Simmer	1 hour 55 min.	3
Rye, flakes	3	Cereal	1 hour 5 min.	2½
Triticale, berries	3	Simmer	1 hour 45 min.	2½
Wheat, berries	3	Simmer	1 hour 10 min.	2½
Wheat, couscous	1½	Steep	5–10 min.	3
Wheat, cracked	2	Cereal	15 min.	2

Grain (1 cup)	Liquid (cups)	Cooking Method*	Cooking Time**	Yield (cups)
Wheat, flakes	4	Cereal	50–55 min.	2
Wheat, bulgur	2	Steep	15 min.	3

*See Cooking Methods, below.

**Cooking times are approximate.

Cooking Methods

To Simmer: Bring liquid to a boil. Stir in grain. Cover and reduce heat to low. Cook until liquid is absorbed and grain is tender to the bite. Fluff with a fork before serving. Soaking whole grains in liquid overnight in the refrigerator will reduce cooking time.

To Steep: Pour boiling liquid over grain. Cover and let stand until grain is tender.

For Cereal (using meal, grits, or flakes): Combine cold water and grain. Bring to a boil, stirring constantly, over high heat. Reduce temperature to low, cover, and cook to desired consistency. Length of time stored can cause fluctuations in cooking time needed. Always check for doneness five minutes before shortest specified cooking time, and then be prepared to cook it longer than the longest specified time.

Tosca's Journal

Well today was a bit of a kitchen disaster! I made lentil tacos, which were delicious, but no one warned me about the dog thinking it might be her food!

Legumes

Beans, from lentils to cannellini to black beans and pintos, vary in color, taste, and texture. Here are some tips:

Buy a variety of dried beans and store them in airtight glass containers in a cool, dark place; they generally stay fresh for six to twelve months.

Dried beans are best if soaked overnight in cold water before being cooked. The soaking time ensures that the beans will be easier to digest, more nutritious, and cook more evenly.

If you're in a hurry, place the beans in a medium pot and cover with two to three inches of water. Bring the water to a boil and then immediately turn off the heat. Let the covered pot of beans sit (at room temp) for at least 1 hour. Drain off all the liquid and then cook the beans according to the recipe; add herbs to taste.

Canned and jarred beans are also a workable option. Again, always read the label and check the sodium count (you want to keep sodium below 500 mg); many brands are low salt or sodium (and fat!) free.

You can store leftover beans in covered containers in the refrigerator; they will stay fresh for at least four days.

Lentils are a tiny, tasty legume that can add zest and protein to a salad or as a side dish. Lentils are easy to prepare and take much less cooking time than beans because they do not need to be soaked. In 3 cups of water, cook 1 cup of lentils for 25 to 40 minutes (depending on the type).

Preparing and Cooking Beans, Lentils, and other Legumes

1 Cup Dry Beans	Cups of Water	Soak Hours	Traditional Boiling Method (minutes)	Slow Cooker		Pressure Cooker		
				Soaked, Low (hours)	Soaked, High (hours)	Soaked, Natural Release (minutes)	Soaked, Quick Release (minutes)	Unsoaked, Quick Release (minutes)
Aduki/adzuki beans	4	None	50 to 60	6	3	2 to 3	5 to 9	14 to 20
Anasazi beans	2½ to 3	4 to 8	50 to 60			1 to 2	4 to 7	20 to 22
Black beans	4	6 to 8	75 to 90	6 to 8	3	4 to 8	5 to 9	8 to 25
Black-eyed peas	3	None	45 to 60		3½	—	—	10 to 11
Borlotti beans	3	6 to 8	45 to 60			5 to 8	9 to 12	30 to 34
Butter beans	4	10 to 12	60 to 90			1 to 3	4 to 7	12 to 16

1 Cup Dry Beans	Cups of Water	Soak Hours	Traditional Boiling Method (minutes)	Slow Cooker		Pressure Cooker		
				Soaked, Low (hours)	Soaked, High (hours)	Soaked, Natural Release (minutes)	Soaked, Quick Release (minutes)	Unsoaked, Quick Release (minutes)
Calypso beans	3	6 to 8	60 to 90			5 to 8	10 to 12	20 to 25
Canary beans	4	8 to 24	60 to 90					
Cannellini beans	3	6 to 8	60 to 90		3	6 to 8		30 to 40
Channa dal	2.5	0 to 4	45 to 90	7				9 to 11
Corona runner	4	6 to 8	60 to 90					
Cow peas, black-eyed peas	3	None	45 to 60		3½			10 to 11
Cranberry beans	3	6 to 8	45 to 60	8 to 9		5 to 8	9 to 12	30 to 34
Fava beans	3	10 to 12	120 to 180		2½			

1 Cup Dry Beans	Cups of Water	Soak Hours	Traditional Boiling Method (minutes)	Slow Cooker		Pressure Cooker		
				Soaked, Low (hours)	Soaked, High (hours)	Soaked, Natural Release (minutes)	Soaked, Quick Release (minutes)	Unsoaked, Quick Release (minutes)
Flageolet beans	3	4 to 8	120 to 150		3½ to 4			
Garbanzo beans (chickpeas)	4	12 to 24	120 to 150	8 to 12	3½ to 4	9 to 14	13 to 18	30 to 40
Great Northern beans	3½	6 to 8	90 to 120		2½	4 to 8	8 to 12	25 to 30
Kidney beans	3	6 to 8	60 to 90		3	5 to 8	10 to 12	20 to 25
Lentils, Beluga	2	None	15 to 20					
Lentils, French green	2	None	45		2	–	–	10 to 12
Lentils, green or brown	2	None		20	1½ to 2	–	–	–
Lentils, ivory	2	None	20			–	–	–

1 Cup Dry Beans	Cups of Water	Soak Hours	Traditional Boiling Method (minutes)	Slow Cooker		Pressure Cooker		
				Soaked, Low (hours)	Soaked, High (hours)	Soaked, Natural Release (minutes)	Soaked, Quick Release (minutes)	Unsoaked, Quick Release (minutes)
Lentils, red, split	2	None	15 to 20		1½	—	—	4 to 6
Lentils, yellow or golden	2	None	20					4 to 6
Limas, baby	4	8 to 10	50 to 60		2½	2 to 3	5 to 7	12 to 15
Limas, Christmas	4	8 to 10	60 to 90					
Limas, large	4	8 to 10	45 to 60		2	1 to 3	4 to 7	12 to 16
Mung beans	2½	4 to 8	45 to 60					
Navy beans (white, haricot)	3	8 to 10	90 to 120			4 to 8	6 to 8	16 to 25
Peas, dried, whole	6	None	60 to 90			4 to 6	8 to 10	16 to 18

1 Cup Dry Beans	Cups of Water	Soak Hours	Traditional Boiling Method (minutes)	Slow Cooker		Pressure Cooker		
				Soaked, Low (hours)	Soaked, High (hours)	Soaked, Natural Release (minutes)	Soaked, Quick Release (minutes)	Unsoaked, Quick Release (minutes)
Peas, split, green or yellow	4	None	45 to 60		2½	—	—	8 to 15
Pink beans	3	6 to 8	50 to 90		3½	6 to 8		
Pinto beans	3	6 to 8	60 to 90	6	3	1 to 3	4 to 6	22 to 25
Rattlesnake beans	3	6 to 8	45 to 60					
Red beans, small	2	6 to 8	60 to 90		2½			
Rice beans	2	None	30 to 45					
Romano beans	3	4 to 8	45 to 60	8 to 9		5 to 8	9 to 12	30 to 34
Scarlet runner beans	4	10 to 24	180 to 240	9 to 12		8 to 10	12 to 14	17 to 20

1 Cup Dry Beans	Cups of Water	Soak Hours	Traditional Boiling Method (minutes)	Slow Cooker		Pressure Cooker		
				Soaked, Low (hours)	Soaked, High (hours)	Soaked, Natural Release (minutes)	Soaked, Quick Release (minutes)	Unsoaked, Quick Release (minutes)
Small red beans	2	6 to 8	60 to 90		2½			
Soy beans (yellow)	4	12 to 24	120 to 180		4	5 to 8	9 to 12	28 to 35
Soy beans (black)	4	12 to 24	180 to 240			16 to 18	20 to 22	35 to 40

Source: www.delectableplanet.com

Pasta

Cooking pasta made of wheat flour, while very easy, is also treated as an art form, especially in Italy where it was invented. As you will see, I strongly suggest that you stick to eating whole-wheat, organic pasta when possible; whole-wheat pasta has more fiber and less of that starchy carb trigger that many of us count among our hidden foods.

Add a pinch of salt to the water before boiling, as this will help lock in the protein and seal the starch from being released. Use the following general cooking times for one pound of whole-grain pasta—and remember, you can keep cooked pasta in a covered container for several days, adding it to sauce (see the fabulous ragu on page 204) or serving as a side salad "dressed" with grilled veggies and a touch of olive oil.

Whole-grain pasta can take double the cooking time of regular pasta. Regular pasta typically takes 4 to 6 minutes to cook; whole-grain pasta can take 10 to 12 minutes. It takes longer for water to break through the complex protein-fiber networks in whole-grain pasta and be reabsorbed. This is a good thing! Whole-grain pasta also has a chewier texture, making it arduous for people with poor dentition. Overcooking whole-grain pasta will soften the texture, although it leads to further nutrient loss.

Whole-grain pasta is typically higher in fiber than regular pasta, although the amount may vary by manufacturer. The higher fiber content comes from the whole-grain flour, which includes the germ and bran. Two ounces of uncooked whole-wheat pasta contain 5 grams of fiber, whereas the equivalent amount of regular pasta contains 2 grams. Fiber helps to remove cholesterol from your digestive system and slows stomach emptying, so you feel fuller longer after a meal. Fiber also helps conquer constipation.

Whole-grain pasta and regular pasta have similar amounts of protein. Two ounces of uncooked whole-wheat pasta contain 8 grams of protein, and 2 ounces of uncooked regular pasta contain 7 grams of protein. Protein is important for cell repair and turnover, and for normal growth and development.

Vegetables

As I mentioned above, I suggest staying away from canned vegetables; if you don't have access to fresh organic veggies, the next best option is frozen—but still try for organic. It's also helpful to buy what's in season: you probably won't find fresh, tasty corn in February, but you will find delicious Brussels sprouts! Think like a farmer when considering your menu and meal plans! What the farmer has harvested that month is not only at its nutritional peak, it's often cheaper because it is so abundant.

You have several cooking options:

Steaming veggies or eating them raw retains the most nutrients.

Blanching is also a good option. To blanch, boil the vegetables in a little water for a very short time (around 2 minutes). Then plunge in a cold water bath.

Lightly sautéing over high heat (you need a good-quality pan for this) in a teaspoon of olive or coconut oil is another quick, delicious technique.

Grilling, roasting, and broiling are also great ways to cook vegetables.

Fish and Meats

You may be excited and relieved that so much fish, chicken, turkey, and lean beef are included in the Start Here plan. This is for both your enjoyment and your health. Again, it's best to purchase meats and fish that are organically raised or wild-caught; they will be cleaner and contain fewer preservatives and/or chemicals.

The key to eating these lean proteins is to enjoy them in moderation. Think of your baby step plate and your healthy portion sizes. Your steak should not be draped over half of your plate and falling over the sides.

Cooking options include:

Grilling
Roasting
Slow-cooking
Baking

Cooking times for meat, poultry, and fish vary a great deal, depending on the size of the portion and the cooking method. In general, it's safe to use a meat thermometer as a guide when roasting meat; grill meat on each side for 15 to 20 minutes, depending on how well done you like your meat. Poultry is generally roasted for 15 minutes per pound. When sautéing or grilling chicken breasts, however, a general rule of thumb is 12 minutes per side. Fish cooks much more quickly: a tuna, halibut, or swordfish steak requires approximately 8 minutes per side, whether it is grilled, pan sautéed, or broiled. A filet of sole (or other thin piece of white fish) cooks even more quickly: about 4 minutes per side.

As you move on to the next chapter, which is filled with four weeks (that's twenty-eight days!) of delicious meal plans, know that you can make many substitutions and adjustments according to your tastes, preferences, and the season. As you become familiar with your Start Here plan, remember to stay flexible and openhearted. You don't want to close a door without giving something a try! As your palate becomes newly accustomed to the flavors of nutrient-dense, whole, natural foods, you will be surprised at how delightful food tastes again.

7

Start Here Meal Plans to Enjoy

The Start Here approach is founded upon its ease, gentleness, and simplicity. I don't want you to get stuck overthinking what you are going to eat each day. I want you to realize that you have options and the freedom to expand your palate and your horizons—within healthy limits, of course! If that freedom includes eating the same thing for breakfast for the next twenty-eight days, that is fine, too.

With that in mind, I have designed a four-week, twenty-eight-day meal plan so you don't have to think; you can just eat and enjoy! I have assembled some healthy breakfast suggestions that will pump you up before you move your body, head to work, or perform any other activities you have planned. Baby step snacks are also well-rounded to keep you feeling balanced and not too hungry, so that you can enjoy your meals and not be triggered to overeat. When I designed the lunches I kept things simple and easy so that they require minimal—if any—prep time. I know most of you, myself included, eat lunch on the go—at our desks, standing in the kitchen, or in our cars, so our food must be portable and uncomplicated.

The dinners are also simple but tend to be a bit heartier. They can easily be eaten for breakfast or lunch, as well. Regardless of what foods you are eliminating in step 2, you still need to pay attention to what's on your plate. These suggestions are just that—suggestions—but do keep in mind all that you've been learning about replating!

Some dieters really enjoy following a meal plan: it helps them shop and prepare their meals two or three days ahead of time. But I know that some of you like to make Start Here your own, so there is plenty of room to adjust the foods that you eat, while still keeping your choices healthy and maximizing your weight loss. Remember, your weight and health are 80 percent tied to the foods you eat! So when planning your meals, make Start Here healthy choices!

Review Your Food Groups
(page 76 in Chapter 4)

ENJOY IN MODERATION

- Protein that is low in negative fats—this includes lean well-sourced grass-fed meats, poultry, seafood, and fermented tofu (tempeh).
- Complex carbohydrates high in fiber—eat whole grains, fruits, and vegetables, with an emphasis on leafy greens.
- Legumes, such as beans and lentils—a mix of complex carbs and protein, these are also high in fiber. They pack a nutrient-rich punch without the fat of meat. Presoak for optimal nutrient value.
- Fats with the proper balance of omega-3, -6, and -9 fatty acids and no trans fats—these include olive oil, coconut oil, fish oil, and nuts and seeds and their oils.

LIMIT

- Simple carbohydrates—these carbohydrates contain high starch and/or sugar and are low in fiber. Found in breads, pastas, rice, potatoes, and sweets.

- Dairy—dairy products, such as milk, cheese, and yogurt, are a good source of protein. Better to eat full, healthy fats but in moderation, plain varieties rather than those loaded with sugar. Cheese should be limited.
- Hydrogenated or trans fats—these fats don't exist in nature; they are man-made and are proven to cause heart disease, cancer, and other serious health conditions and complications.

Tosca's Journal

It's time to celebrate! It's been one entire year of eating clean! With no hidden foods in sight!

Food Tips to Keep in Mind

- Salad dressing: When it comes to dressing your salads, use your best judgment. When out at restaurants, always ask for the dressing on the side, or you can expect lettuce drowning in it. You need just a bit for flavor, so experiment with different bottled dressings, or make your own with a dash of a good olive oil and balsamic or rice wine vinegar. And keep in mind that some oil is necessary to help absorb the nutrients locked in salad greens and vegetables.
- Butter: Use butter in moderate amounts, and buy it unsalted and organic.
- Caffeine: Stay moderate with your caffeine intake (one or two cups of coffee or tea a day), and if drinking dairy in coffee or tea, use cow, almond, rice, or coconut milk.

- Salt: Be mindful of added salt. You know by now that one of the dangers of processed foods, apart from the chemicals and fat lurking within, is the high sodium content. Sodium, one mineral ingredient of salt, has been linked to hypertension and weight gain because it's an appetite stimulant. So please don't add salt to your foods, and if you need a sprinkle, keep it very moderate. I recommend using unrefined sea salt as it contains many necessary minerals, electrolytes, and trace elements.
- No sugar alternatives, fake sugars, or refined white table sugars fit in the Start Here plan. Clean the palate by avoiding all of these and retrain your palate for the taste of sugar. I recommend using raw, natural honey, palm sugar, coconut sugar, maple syrup, or molasses instead. But limit these as well. You don't need much of nature's super-concentrated sweet food.
- Make food for more than one meal—it saves time and money.
- Eat seasonally for the lowest prices and highest nutritional value.

Replating Reminders!

As you peruse the meal plans below, keep your journal handy. You may be inspired by my suggestions and come up with your own. Keep in mind that you always want to include some kind of protein and/or fiber in each snack or meal—either will lower the impact of carbs and sugar on your blood sugar so you feel more in balance. It's also best to enjoy dairy in moderation; dairy contains fat and sodium as well as protein. Hard cheese (e.g., Parmesan, Romano; *not* string or manufactured cheese) has less fat; goat cheese is also good.

Consider portions right from the start. What is on your plate? Is there so much food that you won't be able to eat it without having to undo your pants? Could it feed two or more people? Consider dividing your plate into smaller portions before you eat, placing the extra in small meal-appropriate containers, and storing it for your next meal or snack!

Always accompany a snack or meal with water! Water will flush your body of toxins, move along the digestive process, and keep you hydrated for your best health. If water seems boring, remember, you can lightly flavor it with lemon or cucumber to make it a little more interesting.

Week 1
Indicates recipe included in Chapter 10

Day 1

Breakfast
*Pancakes; water and coffee or tea

Snack
Fruit smoothie with yogurt; water

Lunch
Green salad with grilled chicken; water

Dinner
*Whole Roasted Chicken with Natural Pan Gravy and steamed and mixed vegetables; water

Day 2

Breakfast

*Goat Cheese and Chive Omelet; water and coffee or tea

Snack

Handful of raw almonds and a banana or an apple; water

Lunch

*Quinoa Black Bean Burger; side of fruit salad; water

Dinner

Grilled tuna; side of tomato salad; side of broccoli rabe;
water or herbal tea

Day 3

Breakfast

Fruit smoothie with 1 scoop protein powder; water and
coffee or tea

Snack

Yogurt with trail mix; water

Lunch

Greek salad of romaine lettuce, olives, tomatoes, red onion,
and feta cheese, topped with 1 tablespoon of red wine vinegar
and olive oil, or bottled dressing of your choice; water

Dinner

Grilled salmon, chicken, or shrimp with rice pilaf and a side of
grilled or steamed asparagus; water

Day 4

Breakfast

Peanut (or other nut butter) on Ezekiel or other multigrain
bread or toast; water

Snack

Apple; cottage cheese; water

Lunch

Whole-wheat pita stuffed with hummus, peppers,
tomatoes; water

Dinner

Roasted turkey breast; steamed green beans;
brown rice; water

Day 5

Breakfast

*Apple Cinnamon Oatmeal; water and coffee or tea

Snack

Celery sticks with a dollop of nut butter or cottage cheese;
water

Lunch

Leftover turkey open-faced sandwich on Ezekiel toast with side of unsweetened cranberry relish; water

Dinner

*Peanut Noodles with Chicken and Vegetables; water

Day 6

Breakfast

Two hard-boiled eggs; 1 banana; water

Snack

½ cup red grapes or trail mix (almonds, cashews, dried unsweetened cranberries, raisins); water

Lunch

½ can water-packed tuna with squeeze of lemon; side of tomato salad; water

Dinner

*Taco Night!

Day 7

Breakfast

2 slices of Ezekiel toast with a dollop of nut butter; water

Snack

Grapes, chopped watermelon, pineapple, or cantaloupe
topped with walnuts and a squeeze of fresh lemon; water

Lunch

*Hawaiian Chicken Burger; water

Dinner

*Lemon and Herb Crusted Cod with *Jojo Potatoes; side of
steamed broccoli; water

Week 2

Day 8

Breakfast

*Breakfast Sausage with side of fruit of your choice; water
and coffee or tea

Snack

Apple slices with nut butter; water

Lunch

*Pesto Vegetable and Garbanzo Bean Salad; water

Dinner

*One-Skillet Sweet and Sour Chicken with
steamed broccoli; water

Day 9

Breakfast
*Apple Cinnamon Oatmeal; water

Snack
Handful of almonds; water

Lunch
*Fast-Food Lunch; water

Dinner
*Sloppy Joe Sandwiches; water

Day 10

Breakfast
*Egg 'n' Muffin Breakfast Sandwich; water

Snack
1 slice of Ezekiel toast; water

Lunch
*Mandarin Shrimp Salad; water

Dinner
*Italian Ragu with pasta or rice; water

Day 11

Breakfast
*Egg 'n' Muffin Breakfast Sandwich; water and coffee or tea

Snack
Grapefruit with side of nonfat yogurt and handful
of almonds; water

Lunch
*Greek Pasta Salad; water

Dinner
*Turkey and Brown Rice Patties with side green salad; water

Day 12

Breakfast
*Pancakes (for added fiber, add 1 tablespoon wheat germ
to the batter); water

Snack
Fruit smoothie with yogurt; add a shot of wheatgrass juice
or soy milk; water

Lunch
*Tuna and White Bean Salad Open-Faced Sandwiches; water

Dinner
*Corned Beef with Cabbage, Potatoes, and Root Vegetables;
water

Day 13

Breakfast
*Apple Cinnamon Oatmeal with ¼ cup raisins; water
and coffee or tea

Snack
Fruit smoothie with yogurt; add a shot of protein powder;
water

Lunch
½ can water-packed tuna, with a squeeze of lemon; side of
green salad; water

Dinner
*Whole Roasted Chicken with Natural Pan Gravy dinner with
side of brown rice or quinoa; water

Day 14

Breakfast
2 slices of Ezekiel toast with butter or nut butter; water
and coffee or tea

Snack
1 pear plus sliced leftover roasted chicken; water

Lunch
*Fast-Food Lunch; water

Dinner

Breakfast for dinner: breakfast quesadillas (2 scrambled eggs,
1 tablespoon Monterey Jack cheese, scallions, tomato salsa,
avocado in a whole-wheat tortilla); water

Week 3

Day 15

Breakfast
*Pancakes; water

Snack
Nonfat yogurt with granola; water

Lunch
Green salad with nuts, cranberries, and orange slices (add
sprouts or peppers and avocado if you wish), with
1 tablespoon dressing of your choice; water

Dinner
*Spicy Shrimp and Sausage Gumbo; water

Day 16

Breakfast
*Egg 'n' Muffin Breakfast Sandwich; water

Snack
Good-quality olives, raw almonds, and chunks of very old
Parmesan cheese; water

Lunch
* Quinoa Black Bean Burgers, chicken, or turkey burger
without the bun with a side of green salad; water

Dinner
*Italian Ragu—over pasta, quinoa, or brown rice;
side of green salad; water

Day 17

Breakfast
*Apple Cinnamon Oatmeal; water

Snack
Pineapple chunks and cottage cheese (substitute yogurt if
you don't like cottage cheese); water

Lunch
*Mandarin Shrimp Salad; water

Dinner
*Taco Night!

Day 18

Breakfast

*Pancakes; water and coffee or tea

Snack

Celery sticks with roasted turkey or grilled chicken; water

Lunch

*Hawaiian Chicken Burger; water

Snack

Handful of walnuts or almonds with piece of fruit; water

Dinner

Stir-fry vegetable medley (broccoli and carrots, zucchini and yellow squash, or red, yellow, and orange peppers) over brown rice or quinoa with a side of green salad; water

Day 19

Breakfast

*Goat Cheese and Chive Omelet; water and coffee or tea

Snack

Apple or other crunchy fruit with handful of almonds; water

Lunch

* Quinoa Black Bean Burgers or a fresh turkey or chicken burger and side of fruit salad; water

Dinner

Pasta primavera—pasta of your choice with fresh seasonal vegetables; experiment with combinations, such as squash, peppers, and onions, or canned tomato sauce, eggplant, and broccoli; water

Day 20

Breakfast

1 cup low-fat yogurt with ⅓ cup granola; water

Snack

Banana; water

Lunch

*Greek Pasta Salad; water

Dinner

*Pepper Pot Soup; water

Week 4

Day 21

Breakfast

*Apple Cinnamon Oatmeal with 1 tablespoon honey; water

Snack

Fruit smoothie with protein powder; water

Lunch

*Tuna and White Bean Salad Open-Faced Sandwiches; water

Dinner

*Hawaiian Chicken Burger with side of *Curry Roasted
Cauliflower; water

Day 22

Breakfast

*Breakfast Sausage; water

Snack

½ cup red grapes with handful of walnuts or cashews; water

Lunch

*Mandarin Shrimp Salad; water

Dinner

*Sloppy Joe Sandwiches; water

Day 23

Breakfast

2 slices of Ezekiel toast with unsalted butter; water

Snack

Fruit smoothie with protein powder; water

Lunch
*Pesto Vegetable and Garbanzo Bean Salad; water

Dinner
*Peanut Noodles with Chicken and Vegetables; water

Day 24

Breakfast
Grain cereal with 1 cup low-fat milk and ⅓ cup berries; water

Snack
Apple slices with nut butter; water

Lunch
*Pepper Pot Soup; water

Dinner
Roast turkey with a side of green beans and ½ sweet potato;
water

Day 25

Breakfast
Granola and low-fat yogurt; water and coffee or tea

Snack
Handful of almonds; ½ grapefruit; water

Lunch
*Fast-Food Lunch; water

Dinner
*Quinoa Black Bean Burgers with side of *Roasted Garlic Mashed Potatoes; water

Day 26

Breakfast
*Apple Cinnamon Oatmeal with ¼ cup raisins; water

Snack
1 slice of Ezekiel toast with nut butter; banana; water

Lunch
Nonfat cottage cheese with berries; water

Dinner
*Italian Ragu over pasta, quinoa, or brown rice; side of green salad; water

Day 27

Breakfast
*Egg 'n' Muffin Sandwich; water and coffee or tea

Snack
Apple slices dipped in nonfat yogurt; water

Lunch
Leftover pasta with side of green salad; water

Snack
Sliced cucumbers and carrots with side of hummus; water

Dinner
*Spicy Shrimp and Sausage Gumbo; water

Day 28

Breakfast
Fruit smoothie with protein powder; water

Snack
Celery sticks with hummus; ½ apple; water

Lunch
*Tuna and White Bean Salad Open-Faced Sandwich; water

Snack
Trail mix with an apple or pear; water

Dinner
*Corned Beef with Cabbage, Potatoes,
and Root Vegetables; water

I hope you find delicious favorites and creative inspiration from these suggested meal plans. And keep in mind, these are not your only options! I encourage you to mix and match and try many new combinations from your Start Here grocery list.

These meal plans are a perfect accompaniment to what follows: twenty-eight days of fabulous, easy, and familiar ways to add movement to your life!

8

Moving a Little: Week by Week

Moving a little is your easy, gentle opportunity to introduce exercise into your life—the Start Here way. Although some of you may have not moved or exerted yourselves physically for months or even years, these four seven-week plans are completely doable—regardless of your size, weight, or (former!) athletic ability.

The integration of daily physical activity into your life will maximize your weight loss, make you think more clearly, and reenergize you. You don't have to overhaul your life or radically change your routines to do these movements; they are meant to be familiar. They also work. The week-by-week plan that follows will show you how to integrate the activities in ways that work for you—whether you want to spread out your mini-sessions three times a day, twice a day, or do them all at once. You can also decide when to exercise. Some people like to wake up, have a simple breakfast, and do their exercise. This is my preference. Other people like working out in the middle of the day; instead of sitting down for a long lunch, they use the midday break to fit in their exercise. Still others feel they benefit most from spreading out their exercise in three different periods: early in the day, midday, and then again after work (or before dinner). It's up to you!

The movements are designed to work your entire body not in separate parts but as a whole—which is the way our bodies are meant to move! To breathe deeply and use our bodies is to feel fully human and fully alive. You will find ways to improve your stamina through cardio, your strength through muscle toning, your agility and stability through making your joints more stable, and your posture by connecting to your core.

Now let's start moving!

How the Weeks Work

Weeks 1 and 2 represent the beginner level, offering minimal challenge as you figure out the best ways to integrate these activities into your daily life. Weeks 3 and 4 increase the duration and frequency, offering moderate challenge. Weeks 5 and 6 increase the complexity, duration, and frequency of your activities even more, and represent the highest level of challenge in all three ways. You do not have to follow this plan on that exact calendar schedule, however. You might, for instance, spend one or two months doing the activities described in weeks 1 and 2 (beginning challenge) before you move on to the later weeks. You may even find that you want to alternate the style from week to week, especially if you've been traveling.

I've also balanced the day-by-day selections to include both indoor and outdoor activities, so that you can mix and match depending on your weather or the general climate where you live, or just how you're feeling on any given day. One goal I encourage is to think about exercise as something that happens all the time no matter what, not just when the kids are at school or when you get home from work on time. You will find a selection of easy indoor activities, including chores around the house, plus outdoor activities such as gardening, walking in your neighborhood, and even playing outside with your kids. Rain or shine, you will have plenty of types of movement from which to choose.

The Start Here exercise plan can work for anyone—whether you are returning to exercise after a twenty-year hiatus, if you've been going to a gym every once in a while, or even if you consider yourself a "weekend warrior" athlete. Making physical activity part of your life is about setting the intention that exercise—regardless of its form—is important to you and your health. It's a priority—it's good for your body and your brain and will help you fight disease and the effects of aging.

So yes, it's great to do thirty or forty or sixty minutes on a treadmill, but think about how you can enhance what you are already doing by mixing up the sorts of exercise to include a good balance of cardio, strengthening, and stretching. If you've already been doing some moderate movement, then you might feel comfortable starting with activities in weeks 4 and 5. The plan is not meant to be a prescription but a guide for helping you integrate physical activity in your daily life and improve your all-over body awareness. I believe when just these two simple goals are met, you will have reached success!

Tosca's Journal

Note to self: You are not weak, you are wonderful. You are not fat, you are fabulous. You are not bad, you are beautiful! Keep believing, Tosca!

Creating Your Schedule

In chapter 5, you began to think about how you want to integrate movement into your daily and weekly life—now it's time to create and commit to your schedule. Using either your journal, a planner, or the same whiteboard you posted in your kitchen for your weekly meal plans, create a day-by-day list of movements. Again, I suggest doing this week by week and revising as you go along. If you map out when and what you are going to do, carving out the time in advance, you dramatically increase the likelihood that you will follow through.

Here are some other issues to consider as you plan your weeks ahead:

Avoid Boredom

Avoid getting bored with certain activities by alternating different movements and creating new combinations. Nothing is more of a turnoff than feeling less than excited about an activity! So play with your schedule and challenge yourself to try new activities. Like your mother used to tell you, "take just one bite," try a new activity "just once"—who knows, you may just find you enjoy gardening!

Pay Attention to How You Feel

Check in with how you are feeling. Are you more tired than usual? Have you been drinking enough water? Getting enough sleep? Any kind of exercise will help create energy in your body, but that doesn't mean you don't get fatigued. Make sure you plan for some restorative time to help your muscles relax.

Treat Any Soreness

If your body is sore, don't ignore it. Treat any soreness with lots of water, rest, and Epsom salt soaks. Soreness is a good thing if you treat it regularly, but if your muscles get too tired or you let yourself get too dehydrated, then the soreness may lead to cramps and possibly muscle spasms.

Cue into Posture

Your posture is more than just the backbone of your body. Remember the tips I offered in chapter 5 about pushing your body into your feet? And using your abdominal muscles to strengthen your core? This kind of body awareness not only brings intention to any physical activity you engage in, but it also improves your posture. Good posture is the foundation of being able to move more fluidly throughout the day, with fewer aches and pains.

Mix It Up!

As you create your schedule, remember to mix cardio, strength, and stretching—either in combination on one day or by rotating through the types of activity throughout the week. Remember, your body responds best when it gets all these forms of exercise.

Be Patient with Yourself

As you begin your week, you may feel more tired than you thought, or you may encounter discouraging feelings. Be patient with yourself. Becoming active after being sedentary in your habits for a long time can be quite a shock to the system! So as important as it is to challenge yourself and commit to your schedule, it's also important to pay attention to how you feel. If the suggested three-tiered layout doesn't work well for you, then stick to the movements described in weeks 1 and 2. I trust that when you are ready to move on to more challenge, you will know it!

Weeks 1-2: Beginning Challenge

Week 1 asks you to incorporate fifteen to twenty minutes of activity at least once, preferably twice per day, for four or five days a week. The combinations are designed to get your arms, legs, and core moving, while gently including cardio.

Day 1

Early morning or midday: 15–20 minutes (indoors)
Sweep floors (10 minutes)
Vacuum while holding stomach in (10 minutes)

Late afternoon or early evening: 15–20 minutes (outdoors)
Take an extra trip to the mailbox (5 minutes)
Walk to the end of your driveway or up your block
   (10–15 minutes)

Day 2

Early morning or midday (indoors): 15–20 minutes
Wash the dishes by hand (10 minutes)
Wash down the refrigerator (10 minutes)

Late afternoon or evening (indoors): 15–20 minutes
Climb up and down a flight of stairs twice (10 minutes)
Arm extensions (see pages 93–95; 10 minutes)

Day 3

Early morning or midday (outdoors): 15–20 minutes
Push a stroller or walker up the street, driveway, or
   block (20 minutes)

Late afternoon or early evening (indoors): 15 minutes
Put laundry away piece by piece (15 minutes)

Day 4

Early morning or midday (outdoors): 30–40 minutes
Vacuum car (15–20 minutes)
Wash car windows (15–20 minutes)

Day 5*

Early morning or midday (indoors): 30–40 minutes
Clean out closets (20 minutes)
Do calf raises on steps (10–20 minutes)

Afternoon or early evening (indoors): 10 minutes
Lift feet up and down, keep knee bent at right angle,
    from a seated position

* Optional

Additional Weeks 1–2 Challenge Movements:

Dust the tops of windows
Wash the windows of your house or apartment
Lift your legs up and down while seated, holding in
    stomach muscles
Walk up and down stairs twice, flexing your wrists
Clean out your pantry and cupboards
Walk the driveway or office corridor
Do gentle twists from a standing position
Lie on the floor and do chin tucks
Lie on the floor, tuck knees, and twist to the side
Lift your legs up and down while standing, holding in
    stomach muscles

Weeks 3-4: Moderate Challenge

Weeks 3-4 movements ask you to add one extra day of activity and increase your duration by five to ten minutes. The movements are slightly more challenging in their cardio and strengthening capacity, and you will be incorporating more stretching. Keep in mind that you can shift the times when you exercise as well as the combinations, but try to balance out the cardio, strengthening, and stretching movements from day to day, workout to workout.

Day 1

Early morning or midday (outdoors): 20–25 minutes
Walk the block around your home or office
(20–25 minutes)

Afternoon or evening (indoors): 15–20 minutes
Sit on the edge of your bed and raise your arms (see arm extensions, pages 93–95; 15–20 minutes)

Day 2

Early morning or midday (indoors): 45 minutes
Paint a piece of furniture (30 minutes)
Clean the tub (15 minutes)

Afternoon or evening (indoors): 20–30 minutes
Move the furniture of 2-3 rooms and vacuum floors
completely (20–30 minutes)

Day 3

Early morning or midday (outdoors): 35–45 minutes
Push a grocery cart through the store 3-4 times
  (20–30 minutes)
Walk to the mailbox at the end of your street and back
  twice (15 minutes)

Afternoon or evening (indoors): 30 minutes
Sit on edge of bed and do leg lifts (see leg lifts, pages
  93–95; 15 minutes)
Sit on edge of bed and do arm extensions (see arm
  extensions, pages 93–95; 15 minutes)

Day 4

Early morning or midday (outdoors): 30 minutes
Plant flowers or pick weeds in garden (30 minutes)

Afternoon or evening (indoors): 30 minutes
Clean tub (15 minutes)
While sitting at your desk, in your car, or on the
  subway, pull in your stomach muscles (15 minutes)

Day 5

Early morning or midday (outdoors): 30 minutes
Walk when you'd usually take a taxi or bus
  (20–30 minutes)

Afternoon: 30 minutes

Walk the mall with a friend (30 minutes)

Day 6*

Early morning or midday (outdoors): 45–60 minutes

Go apple picking, visit a museum, or take a tour
of a historic site

* Optional

Additional Weeks 3–4 Challenge Movements:

Water aerobics or swimming

Play with your kids

Rake the lawn

Wash your car

Ride your bike

Dance (at home or in a class)

Fencing

Treadmill

Weeks 5-6: High Challenge

This third level of movement continues to raise your exertion level and increases the frequency and duration of activities. However, keep in mind you can stick to doing your activities twice a day, or add a third session. This is entirely up to your personal preference and schedule. You may enjoy exercising in short but frequent bursts, splitting up your activities at the beginning and end of the day, or you may prefer to do it all at once—for a sustained amount of time.

Day 1

Early morning: 25 minutes

Walk up and down stairs 3–4 times (10 minutes)

Lying on your bed on your back or stomach, do 10
scissor kicks, (repeat for 5–10 minutes)

From a standing position, touch your toes (5 minutes)

Noon or midday: 15–20 minutes

Walk around your block from office or home
(15–20 minutes)

Afternoon or evening: 15 minutes

Neck rolls (15 minutes)

Day 2

Early morning: 25 minutes

Clean out garage or storage unit (25 minutes)

Noon or midday: 20–25 minutes

Arm extensions (10 minutes)

Leg extensions (10 minutes)

Neck rolls (5 minutes)

Afternoon or evening: 15 minutes

Walk your block or go to the mall with a friend
(15 minutes)

Day 3

Early morning: 30 minutes

From your bed, do twists (10 minutes)

From a standing position, raise your knees (10 minutes)

From a standing position, touch your toes (10 minutes)

Easy Stretch—see page 170 (10 minutes)

Noon or midday: 30 minutes

Treadmill* (15 minutes)

Bike* (15 minutes)

* If you don't have access to a stationary bike or a treadmill, replace both with 30 minutes of walking. Or climb the stairs at your house repeatedly.

Day 4

Early morning: 35–45 minutes

Take a walk with friend in park or woods

   (25-30 minutes)

Easy Stretch—see page 170 (10-15 minutes)

Noon or midday: 10–15 minutes

Arm lifts with cans (10-15 minutes)

Day 5

Early morning: 30 minutes

Push a stroller or walker around the block (20 minutes)

Arm extensions (10 minutes)

Noon or midday: 20 minutes

Walk the stairs (10 minutes)

Neck rolls (10 minutes)

Evening: 25 minutes

Arm extensions (10 minutes)

Leg extensions (10 minutes)

Neck rolls (5 minutes)

Day 6*

Early morning: 35–45 minutes

Treadmill or stationary bike (20–25 minutes)

Arm extensions (10 minutes)

Leg lifts (10 minutes)

Noon or midday: 10 minutes

Easy Stretch—see page 170 (10 minutes)

* Optional

Additional Weeks 5–6 Challenge Movements:

Zumba

Pilates

Core workout

Elliptical machine

StairMaster

Cycling

Tennis

Swimming

Circuit or interval training

Jog or run

Cross Fit

Endurance events

Bonus Week: Highest Challenge

The six-week cycle described above will improve your strength, agility, and overall physical stamina. The exercises listed for the bonus week are designed to maximize your physical challenge. You may want to alternate a tough week with a less demanding week, giving yourself a challenge and then backing off for a rest. Keep in mind that the movements designed in this week are meant for those who have been exercising frequently for a number of months and have built up strength, endurance, and flexibility. But as you move through the plan, you may just want to test the water! So come on in—it's fabulous!

Day 1

Early morning: 20 minutes
Walk/run around neighborhood or on treadmill
(15–20 minutes)

Afternoon or evening: 40 minutes
Arm extensions (10 minutes)

Neck rolls (10 minutes)

Inner thigh squeeze (10 minutes)

Raise knees (10 minutes)

Day 2

Early morning: 30–40 minutes
Walk/run on treadmill (15 minutes)

Stationary bike or road bike (15–20 minutes)

Afternoon or evening: 20 minutes

Arm weights from prone position—biceps curls,
overhead lat pulls, and goal posts—see page 170 for
description (15 minutes)

Easy Stretch (5–10 minutes)

Day 3

Early morning: 35–45 minutes

Treadmill or stationary bike (20–25 minutes)

Arm weights (10 minutes)

Squats (10 minutes)

Afternoon or evening:15 minutes

Easy Stretch, Neck rolls (15 minutes)

Day 4

Early morning: 35–45 minutes

Take a run/walk with a friend in the park or woods
(25–30 minutes)

Easy Stretch (10–15 minutes)

Afternoon or evening: 15–20 minutes

Swim (20-35 minutes)

Arm weights—or use your cans! (10 minutes)

Leg lifts (10 minutes)

Day 5

Early morning: 30 minutes

Quick run/walk in neighborhood (20 minutes)

Squats (5 minutes)

Triceps dips (5 minutes)

Crunches (5 minutes)

Afternoon or evening: 30–45 minutes

Easy Stretch, Neck rolls

Day 6*

Early morning: 30–40 minutes

Swim (20–35 minutes)

Bike (15–20 minutes)

Afternoon or evening: 20 minutes

Arm weights (15 minutes)

Easy Stretch (15 minutes)

* Optional

Additional Bonus Week Challenge Movements:

Spin class or cycle

Jump rope

Kickboxing

Tennis

Rowing machine

Squash

Circuit training with weights

Interval training

Arm Extensions: Stretch arms overhead, to the side in T position, and bring them back to your sides. (10x)

Arm Weights:

Biceps Curls: With small 2- to 3-pound weights, keep elbows at sides, and curl your forearms toward your body. (10x)

Goal Posts: Lie on floor mat, place arms out to side, and bend them at right angle (forming "goal posts"); with small 2- to 3-pound weights, lift bent arms toward ceiling. (10x)

Overhead Lat Pulls: Lie on floor mat, and with 2- to 3-pound light weights, extend your arms overhead; pressing back and stomach into the floor, raise and lower the weights off floor to above your face. (10x)

Easy Stretch: Lie on floor mat, stretch arms out to side in T position, pull knees in, and stretch them to one side and then the other.

Inner Thigh Squeeze: Lie on your back with legs out straight; place a 7″ soft ball or pillow between your legs, and squeeze your legs together, hold for 5 seconds, and release. (10x)

Knee Raises: From a standing or seated position, lift bent knee toward the ceiling, pulling in stomach as you raise leg. (10x)

Leg Lifts: On floor mat, straighten leg and lift, while pressing stomach muscles into floor; lift leg only as high as you can maintain a flat back. (10x)

Neck Rolls: Lie on floor mat, press your back into floor and gently turn your neck to right, then left, while keeping shoulders on floor.

9

A Constant in Your Life:

Troubleshooting Disruptions and
Staying on Course

"I never have a problem eating in a healthy way when nothing is going on in my life—the problem is that never happens!"

"It's so hard for me to balance what my family wants to eat and still stick to a clean diet. How do I make it work?"

"I am totally committed to staying away from my hidden foods during my normal life. But what about vacation, travel, and holidays? What do I do then?"

All these voices from the field echo one of the biggest challenges of any diet or eating plan: How do you stay on track and organized in a less than perfect world? Throughout this book we've talked about how to stay in touch with how you feel, the emotional situations that can get you off course, and the triggers that may send you flying back to your hidden foods. But old habits die hard, so this chapter is dedicated to showing you how easily you can make empowering decisions—no matter what is going on in your life.

Mobilize Your Support

Before going into all the ways your new healthy lifestyle can be disrupted, I want to remind you of all the tools you have to support your goals, reinforce your commitment, and ready yourself for the inevitable interruptions and challenges in your daily life.

Since taking the three Start Here steps, you've been keeping a record of your thoughts and feelings, reminding yourself of both your near and far goals; integrated at least fifteen to twenty minutes of physical activity into your daily routine; and, most important, replated your meals and snacks so that they maximize your health and your weight loss.

Whether you have out-of-town guests, are in the middle of a stressful work cycle, are enduring some other disruptive situation, or just balancing your daily life, all of these steps can be reinforced if you mobilize support—from both inside and outside yourself. Here's how:

- Prepare the people in your life: your family, friends, and co-workers will be sure to notice the changes you are making in every aspect of your life, so why not tell them explicitly? The people in your life should know how important your Start Here steps are to you.
- Prepare yourself for people who will try to derail you during the process. Sometimes these are family or friends living with you who are frightened about your perceived changes. They may become angry and attempt to stop you in your tracks. Often these people do this not intentionally or in a mean-spirited way, but simply because they are responding in fear to the idea that you are changing. You don't have to accept their sabotaging efforts, but you may have to let them know you are committed to your process and need their positive support.
- Invite a friend to join you. We are never alone in our circum-

stances, and this applies to the desire and need to change one's life through eating in a more healthy way. Think of someone in your life you are in touch with regularly and make a pact to do some or all of the steps together. If this person lives in a different town or state, you can set up regular Skype or telephone calls to exchange notes, report on progress or obstacles, or share triumphs.

- Share your experience with all of us at Kitchen Table (www.toscareno.com). You can also gain support through our Start Here Twitter and Facebook pages. Sharing your experience, reading the experiences of others, and responding will help reinforce your goals and keep you on track.

- Go one-on-one with Tosca. Believe it or not, I do respond to emails from individual clients. I also travel to many conferences where I can engage one-on-one or in small groups. It is my sincere hope that I continue to do so as more and more join the Start Here family. So please, reach out to me via email and let me hear about your experience!

Mood Swings

✴ Elated, unstable, emotional, uncertain, excited—this may describe how you've been feeling these past weeks and months as you remove your hidden foods and clean up your diet. Many clients have described intense and frequent shifts in their moods as they drop foods and old habits that have literally blocked them from feeling. With these barricades removed, suddenly myriad feelings rise to the surface: anger, shame, remorse, embarrassment, and fear. These difficult emotions can make us feel very uncomfortable, and understandably so.

Instead of trying to look the other way, look right at those feelings: admit to yourself that you feel sad, angry, or confused. Let those feelings just exist within you, and don't try to hide from them anymore. Then remind yourself of your goals, turn to your goals as affirmations, and take three breaths (inhale, exhale slowly).

Soon, as the days and weeks pass, your feelings will stabilize, righting your emotional ship. You will feel more steady, and you will experience the confidence, clarity, and optimism that come with eating clean.

Tosca's Journal

I don't miss my mood swings anymore. I don't miss the sugar hangover in the morning. The cravings around 3 P.M. I don't miss anything about my hidden foods.

Family Matters

Whether you are single or married, with children or without, staying on track with your goals gets complicated when other people are involved. If you must manage other people's schedules, shop and prepare meals, or even simply eat alongside other people who are not doing Start Here, then it's important that you stay clear and acknowledge that you may be eating differently than others. Different is not bad or less than. Different is not selfish or complicated. Different is just different. You can try saying something like "I really love the abundance of energy I feel when I eat this way," or "I love feeling good about myself when I know I am following my Start Here plan. It makes me want to be a better mother." Remind yourself that you are a work in progress; your total transformation is under way and you are loving the early results. Tell yourself you are in love with the newness taking place in and on you, and you love it more than someone else's negativity. Keep shining your bright light. This leads the way for others to follow. Take a pass on any negative energy; it is not something to respond to.

As I suggest above, if those with whom you live and work are aware of your goals and commitment to eating the Start Here way, then they are more likely to be supportive and not question or criticize. They may even want to taste some of your new, enticing food options! But regardless of whether your family and friends join you, you still need to take some logistical steps to keep things simple.

Here are some tips:

- If you are the preparer of the family meals, try making your own breakfast, lunch, or dinner in advance so that you don't run out of time and end up not doing it.
- Keep your staples on hand—grilled chicken, rice or other grains, hummus, veggies (sautéed, steamed, or grilled), lots of salad fixings!
- Leftovers! If you're the primary chef, then cook enough of your grains, meats, and veggies to last for two or three days. As you will note in many of the recipes, it's easy to double the amounts and store leftovers in the refrigerator.
- Encourage your family to try what you are eating. Since all the foods are clean, tasty, and healthy, someone else is bound to enjoy them, too!
- Sit down and enjoy your meal—alone or with your family. Don't eat standing up or separately; even if you're eating differently, you're still a part of the group!

Travel and Life on the Go

I travel so much that my car virtually drives itself to the airport, so I know how challenging it is to stick to a healthy way of eating. And even when I am in my hometown, I am constantly on the go—rushing from one end of the day to the next. It can feel overwhelming to plan your food at seven in the morning before the day begins!

When I know that I am going to be in transit for a day or two, I make sure I have packed some fresh foods—especially snacks—that will keep me sated until I have a meal. I feel most vulnerable when I get too hungry and I have to hunt down some food; this is when many of us get caught making bad food choices. So instead of reaching for that bag of chips, donut, or candy bar to tide you over, try a simplified version of what I refer to as my "Cooler Concept."

In a small cooler or insulated lunch bag, pack three or four snacks that will keep fresh for several hours:

- Small yogurt
- Two or three pieces of fruit (apple, pear, cut-up watermelon or cantaloupe, chunks of coconut)
- Hard cheese
- Raisin-nut mix (see page 140 for my homemade combination!)

If you are on the road for longer than twenty-four hours, and you want to fill a regular-size cooler with ice packs, consider these healthy snack and light meal options:

- Hard-boiled egg
- Small container of cottage cheese
- Whole-grain wrap with grilled chicken and sliced tomato
- Small container of tunafish
- Fruit smoothie (see page 222 for my quick homemade version!)

It's inevitable that at some point you'll eat out when traveling, and when that happens, just get food you know is safe. Every airport restaurant has a salad, for example. It might not be the very best meal, but it beats French fries, a bag of chips, or candy, and you won't believe how proud of yourself you'll be for making that decision!

If you have to do a lot of driving for extended periods of time, your best investment is one of those coolers you can plug into your car. When I hop into my car for a road trip, my cooler brims with prepared chicken breasts, quinoa salad, hummus and crudités, muesli, dried berries, fresh fruit, and flax crackers. You can keep anything in there that you would in a normal fridge, and it will likely come with an adapter so you can plug it in when you get to your hotel/motel. This may sound like a lot of planning, time, and effort, but once you get into the habit of grilling several chicken breasts for the week, keeping your fridge stocked with fruit and crunchy vegetables like carrots, cucumbers, celery, and red peppers—all of which travel well—you will get so used to having healthy food on hand you will miss it sorely when it is not. Eating to be a Start Here pro can be quite addicting.

The trick is to never go too long without eating. By keeping healthy snacks (see page 176) in your bag, car, or cooler, you can stave off hunger until you get somewhere to enjoy a healthy meal. Eating regular meals at three-hour intervals also means you will keep blood sugar levels steady and your metabolism burning on high, both of which add up to fat loss.

Fast-Food Options

✴ Fast-food restaurants are notorious for their processed, high-fat, high-calorie, enormous-portion-size food nightmares. However, when you are traveling or simply too busy to eat a more leisurely and healthy meal, then it's good to know that most fast-food restaurants offer some reasonably healthy options. Below is a list of the most healthy suggestions at each of these popular spots; you'll notice that most of the offerings involve grilled chicken and salad. This means, avoid the French fries, burgers, and other fried and breaded options!

McDonald's—Asian Chicken Salad (no croutons)

Burger King—Tendergrill Chicken Garden Salad

Wendy's—Mandarin Chicken Salad

Subway—Grilled Chicken Sandwich on whole-wheat bun, open-faced if possible, no sauce

Taco Bell—Chicken Ranch Taco, Fresco Style (no sauce, cheese, or avocado dressing)

Hardee's/Carl's Jr. (the name of the chain in the west)— Charbroiled BBQ Chicken Sandwich (no BBQ sauce)

Sonic—Grilled Chicken Salad (no croutons)

Chick-Fil-A—Chargrilled Chicken Salad—(no croutons)

Jack in the Box—Asian Grilled Chicken Salad

Dining Out: Make Simple Choices

Food is meant to be a pleasure, not just a necessity, and many of us enjoy not only the food but also the experience of dining out at a restaurant. Others of us eat frequently in restaurants due to our work obligations. Regardless of our motivation, ordering at a restaurant can be cumbersome, difficult, and even a bit scary when you feel like there are right and wrong decisions to be made. As one client tweeted,

"How do I stay true to my Start Here plan with all these marvelous choices?"

Here are some simple strategies to stick to when eating at a restaurant:

- Skip the bread! Before even being tempted by the smell of fresh-baked rolls or focaccia, ask the server to remove it or—better yet—not even place it on the table. Somebody once suggested that I ask the waiter to bring out fresh-cut veggies instead, and I was surprised to learn that some restaurants won't charge you for a little plate of celery and carrot sticks instead of bread!

- Peruse the menu and look for dishes that are not fried or breaded or served with a cream sauce.

- If you find a lean meat or fish that you think you might enjoy, ask the server if you may have it prepared without sauce or lightly sautéed.

- When ordering pasta, go with a red sauce or olive oil. The white sauces tend to be butter and/or cream based.

- When your meal is served, use your replating skills to portion off the amount of food you are now accustomed to eating; remember, you can always bring home the leftovers, and get to enjoy the restaurant experience twice!

- Always order a salad with, before, or even after a meal! The greens will help fill you and aid digestion.

- Don't overdo the alcohol. It's tempting to join the crowd and drink more wine or cocktails than you are used to; if you want to enjoy a glass of wine with dinner, limit it to one glass and sip on water throughout your meal.

- Skip dessert or share one for the table. It's hard to avoid delicious desserts at restaurants, but instead of throwing off your body chemistry with a big portion of something sugary, give yourself a bite or two to sate your sweet tooth and then put your fork away.

Holidays and Vacation: Give a Little

Two words come to mind when I think of food and holidays or vacation: relax and indulge. After all, isn't that what we want to get out of our precious time on vacation or during holidays with family and friends? We want to take it easy, get a break from our normal lives, and live a little; we want to give ourselves some well-deserved treats or perhaps indulge in the cuisine of a new locale. So how do you allow this very human need for a break in your regular routine without sabotaging your goals?

You give a little.

Yes—give yourself a little treat during holiday times and on vacation. You will not only enjoy such treats more fully (now that you are eating mindfully!), but you can also trust yourself to be measured in your indulgence. The key is moderation. So how do you keep a healthy balance when it comes to the sweets, baked breads, cocktails, and other sundries that surround us on vacation and during the holidays?

Here are my top tips to enjoy the holiday (or vacation) without paying the consequences:

1. Don't arrive hungry! What does this mean? Pre-eat! I often do this before going to an event, party, or holiday gathering where I can't be sure when the meal will be served or what it will be. If I give myself a healthy snack such as an apple with a dollop of nut butter, a side of hummus with celery or carrots, or even a grilled chicken breast cold from the fridge, then I will arrive at the festivities feeling calm rather

than hungry. It's easier to make smart decisions when you aren't being motivated by a growling stomach, and pre-eating puts you in a position to make good choices, and even indulge a little bit, rather than overindulging in a way you'll regret later.

2. Tackle the buffet. If the luncheon or dinner is a buffet, you will more than likely find some options that fit with your new regime. Scan the buffet table and look for the fresh fruit, vegetables, fish or meats, and grains. Let the veggie or fruit crudités scream "fresh, just-picked goodness." This is your sign they have been prepared from scratch and not doused in oil or sauce. Chilled seafood and pickled vegetables are also good options. Another buffet trick is to select a dessert plate rather than a large dinner plate. You will be less likely to load up Fred Flintstone–style if your plate is small.

   The buffet may be piled high with cheesy, gooey temptations. Stay clear of these. It is difficult to know what ingredients are buried in them, and if a dish looks saucy and gooey, it probably has loads of excess unwanted fat—most of which may not be the good kind.

3. Politely and discreetly portion off what you want to eat. No manner guide insists you provide your hostess with a clean plate; make sure that you compliment the chef on a great meal, but don't feel like you have to eat every bite of it!

4. Be wary of hidden calories. Being aware of where sugar hides in food and drink is a solid technique in the Start Here program. Alcohol is a form of sugar, so just like any sweet, it will trigger a cascade of impacts you are now very familiar with. I occasionally indulge in a glass of wine or a

beer, but I limit myself to one. When I do, I always have a glass of water in the other hand.

5. Gracefully conquer setbacks. Disruptions to our routines are powerful reminders to stay in touch with our near and far goals and how good we feel when we are eating right. But sometimes these reminders are not enough, and we fall off course. When that happens—and believe me, it happens to all of us—we have to trust ourselves and know we can get back on course.

   Maybe it's a one-day affair, maybe it's a week or a month. Things happen in our lives that interrupt our flow, undermine our willpower, and cause us to question our commitments. But you have been developing the inner strength—mental, physical, and emotional—to weather any storm. The first thing you need to do is forgive yourself. Don't waste time beating yourself up for eating a slice of fabulous chocolate cake at your daughter's wedding or drinking three glasses of wine at your niece's bat mitzvah.

6. Reward yourself—without food. Turn to other ways to reward yourself and develop other favorite treats that are not related to food: go to the movies, get your nails done, get a massage, call a friend who lives far away, buy some new workout clothes, treat yourself to a scarf, lipstick, or perfume.

7. Make sure you get enough sleep. A rested brain and body will help you feel more balanced. You will lower the chances of making less-than-ideal choices.

8. Use your mindset techniques (see page 29) to shift your focus from the negative to the positive. Letting your brain and your body rehearse the changes helps to uproot old behaviors and instill the new patterns.

9. Get back to it. No matter how long your slip might have been, know that you can get right back to eating the Start Here way, including your exercise. Just like your muscles have memory, so does your belly. With your body back into its routine, you will feel better in no time!

10

Start Here Recipes

These recipes are absolutely delicious, easy to prepare, and nutritionally optimal as you begin to lose weight and get in shape. Through the recipes, I've noted ways to add more protein or cut down on fat and other nutritional tips. I understand that some days you feel hungrier than others and will want more "heft" to your meal. The more familiar you get with the recipes and the basics, the more obvious your adjustments will be to your own replating strategies. But until that happens, it's better to be safe than sorry. After all this good work, you don't want to trigger any old habits!

Breakfast

Don't skip breakfast! In fact, it's optimal to eat within one hour of waking. All of us wake up with low blood sugar, so it's important to give your body some fuel to jump-start your metabolism and increase your chances of having a day of high energy and clear thinking.

Apple Cinnamon Oatmeal

Prep: 10 minutes   •   Cook: 10 minutes
Yield: 3 cups; two 1½-cup servings or three 1-cup servings

This oatmeal can be made ahead of time and packed in "to go" containers to take with you. Add a scrambled or hard-boiled egg to make a complete breakfast.

1 tablespoon organic unsalted butter
1 apple, cut into ½-inch dice
½ teaspoon cinnamon
1 cup old-fashioned oats
1¾ cups water
Pinch of sea salt
1 tablespoon brown sugar (or step up to
   maple syrup or honey)
1 tablespoon sliced almonds or chopped walnuts (optional)
1 cup milk

In a small pot over moderate heat, melt the butter and add the apple. Cook until softened and golden brown, stirring occasionally, 5 minutes. Stir in the cinnamon to coat. Add the oats, water, and salt. Bring to a simmer and cook for 5 minutes. If the oatmeal gets too thick, add a little more water. Remove from heat, cover, and let stand for 3 minutes. Uncover and stir in the brown sugar. Divide among bowls, top with almonds or walnuts, and pour in the milk. Eat warm.

TNT (Tosca Nutrition Tip)

✻ The almonds, walnuts, and milk help to "lock in" the carbs, so that your blood sugar doesn't spike and you don't trigger carb cravings.

Breakfast Sausage

Prep: 15 minutes   •   Cook: 10 minutes
Yield: 8 patties

Are you too busy in the morning to make breakfast? Here's a solution! Make these the night before, then wrap them individually in plastic wrap or resealable plastic bags. In the morning, just grab a couple out of the fridge and go! You have a healthy instant breakfast on the run.

TNT

✴ The fruit adds fiber to the meat. The apple also adds a sweet but tart flavor, and you get that "full feeling" without the chemicals and fat of regular sausage!

1 teaspoon extra virgin olive oil
¼ yellow or white onion, grated
½ green apple, such as Granny Smith, grated
½ pound lean ground turkey or chicken
½ pound lean ground pork (or step up to all ground chicken
    or turkey to make it lighter in calories and lower in fat)
½ cup bran flakes, crushed (or step up to ¼ cup oat bran
    or wheat germ)
¼ teaspoon poultry seasoning (salt-free)
¼ teaspoon garlic powder
⅛ teaspoon ground nutmeg
½ teaspoon sea salt
¼ teaspoon freshly ground black pepper
Eat-Clean cooking spray

Heat the olive oil in a large skillet over moderate heat. Add the onion and apple and cook until soft, 3 minutes. Remove from heat and allow to cool slightly.

In a large bowl, combine the ground turkey and pork, bran flakes, poultry seasoning, garlic powder, nutmeg, salt, and pepper. Add the cooked onion and apple. Mix the ingredients together well. Shape into 8 patties.

Heat a nonstick skillet over moderate heat and coat with Eat-Clean spray. Add the patties in a single layer and cook until browned, then flip and cook until no longer pink in the center, about 5 minutes.

Cooking Tip: You can also cook the patties in a 350°F oven. To test for doneness, cut one in half. If it's no longer pink, it's ready to eat!

Egg 'n' Muffin Breakfast Sandwich

Prep: 10 minutes • Cook: 5 minutes
Yield: 1 breakfast sandwich

Eat-Clean cooking spray

1 egg

1 whole-grain English muffin

1 teaspoon reduced-fat olive oil mayonnaise
    (drop the mayo to step up this dish)

1 teaspoon prepared mustard

¼ cup alfalfa sprouts

¼ avocado, sliced

2 tomato slices

Sea salt

Freshly ground black pepper

Fill the bottom of an egg poacher with an inch of water and bring to a simmer over medium-high heat. Spray a poaching cup with cooking spray and add the egg to the cup. Cover the pan and cook the egg until the white is set and the yolk is slightly thickened, 3 to 4 minutes. Remove the cup from the poacher and use a knife to gently loosen the edge of the egg from the cup.

Meanwhile, toast the English muffin. Spread the mayonnaise and mustard on half of the muffin. Add the sprouts and place the egg on top. On the other half, layer the avocado and tomato slices. Season the egg and veggies with a pinch of salt and pepper, bring both sides of the muffin together, and enjoy!

Goat Cheese and Chive Omelet

Prep: 5 minutes   •   Cook: 5 minutes
Yield: 1 serving

2 eggs
1 tablespoon whole milk (or step up to
    reduced-fat milk)
Pinch of sea salt and freshly ground black pepper
Eat-Clean cooking spray
1 tablespoon soft goat cheese, such as chèvre
1 tablespoon finely chopped chives or
    scallions (green part only)

In a bowl, whisk together the eggs, milk, and salt and pepper.

Heat an 8-inch nonstick skillet over medium-low heat and spray with cooking spray. Pour the eggs into the skillet and cook until they start to firm up around the edges. Lift up the edges with a rubber spatula to let the eggs run underneath, repeating until the eggs are set. Sprinkle the goat cheese and chives over the top. Using the spatula, fold the omelet in half and slide onto a plate.

Pancakes . . . or Waffles

The batter can be used for either!

Prep: 15 minutes • Cook: 15 minutes
Yield: twelve 5-inch pancakes

½ cup old-fashioned oats
2 cups milk or buttermilk

Dry Ingredients:
1½ cups whole-wheat flour
2 teaspoons baking powder
½ teaspoon baking soda
¼ teaspoon sea salt

Wet Ingredients:
2 eggs
¼ cup brown sugar (or step up to honey)
1 tablespoon extra virgin olive oil or grapeseed oil
½ teaspoon vanilla extract

1 cup frozen or fresh blueberries (optional)
Eat-Clean cooking spray

In a medium bowl, mix together the oats and buttermilk and set aside. In a separate large bowl, sift together the dry ingredients. Stir the wet ingredients into the oat and buttermilk mixture, then add to the dry ingredients. Mix until just moistened. The batter will be lumpy. Gently stir in blueberries, if desired.

Heat a griddle or large nonstick skillet thoroughly over medium-low heat. Spray with Eat-Clean spray.

Pour the batter onto the griddle to make the desired-size pancakes, leaving 1 inch between them. Cook until the batter starts to bubble on top and is dry around the edges. Carefully flip and cook for one more minute. Repeat until all the batter is used.

This batter can also be used to make waffles. Simply cook in a waffle iron sprayed with Eat-Clean spray.

Lunches

Lunch is rarely leisurely for any of us, so you want to make sure you have foods on hand that you can bring to work or are ready to eat out of your fridge if you're home. Again, the key is not to let yourself get too hungry between breakfast and lunch; have a handful of almonds at 10 A.M., or eat half of your sandwich if you feel really hungry. Learn to cue into your real hunger and you will begin to feel more balanced throughout the day. You will also be able to resist the tendency to overeat when you do sit down for a meal.

Fast-Food Lunch

Prep: 5 minutes   •   Cook: 5 minutes
Yield: 1 complete meal

Tip: You can substitute a Turkey and Brown Rice Patty (page 198) for the whole-grain toast or cooked brown rice.

Eat-Clean cooking spray
2 eggs
4 cups lightly packed fresh spinach
1 slice of whole-grain bread, toasted, or
    ½ cup cooked brown rice
1 teaspoon organic unsalted butter
½ tomato, thinly sliced
Sea salt and freshly ground black pepper

Fill the bottom of an egg poacher with an inch of water and bring to a simmer over medium-high heat. Spray 2 poaching cups with Eat-Clean cooking spray and add the eggs. Cover the pan and cook the eggs until the whites are set and the yolks are slightly thickened, 3 minutes. Remove the cups from the poacher and set aside.

Meanwhile, heat a nonstick skillet over medium heat. Add the spinach and a small splash of water. Using tongs, turn the spinach a few times until it wilts. Remove from heat and transfer to a plate. Toast the bread and spread with the butter.

Use a knife to loosen the edges of the eggs from their cups, then slide them onto the toast. Fan out the tomato slices next to the eggs and spinach. Season the eggs with a small pinch of sea salt and black pepper.

Greek Pasta Salad

Prep: 25 minutes   •   Cook: 10 minutes
Yield: ten 2-cup servings

TNT

✳ Add grilled chicken, fish, or other lean, healthy protein to make this a complete meal.

12 ounces multigrain or whole-grain corkscrew pasta (rotini), or similar shape

1 15-ounce can reduced-sodium garbanzo beans, drained and rinsed

10 cups mixed baby greens (or spinach, or any other salad greens you have on hand)

1 red bell pepper, seeded and thinly sliced into 2-inch pieces

1 green bell pepper, seeded and thinly sliced into 2-inch pieces

½ English cucumber, chopped

2 scallions, thinly sliced

½ cup drained, pitted kalamata olives, coarsely chopped

2 cups cherry or grape tomatoes, halved

½ cup crumbled feta (or step up to reduced-fat feta)

¼ cup chopped fresh basil

2 tablespoons finely chopped fresh oregano

Grated zest and juice of 1 large lemon

3 tablespoons red wine vinegar

3 tablespoons extra virgin olive oil

½ teaspoon sea salt

1 teaspoon freshly ground black pepper

Bring a large pot of salted water to boil and cook the pasta according to package directions until tender, but still firm to the bite. Drain well and place in a very large bowl.

Add the garbanzo beans, baby greens, red and green bell peppers, cucumber, scallions, olives, tomatoes, feta, basil, and oregano.

In a small bowl, whisk together the lemon zest and juice, vinegar, olive oil, salt, and pepper.

Pour over the pasta salad and toss to combine.

Pesto Vegetable and Garbanzo Bean Salad

Prep: 20 minutes • Cook: 5 minutes
Yield: 12 cups; six 2-cup main course servings (add chicken or other protein), or twelve 1-cup side dish servings

1 pound asparagus, tough stalks trimmed,
   cut into 2-inch pieces

½ pound broccoli crowns, cut into 2-inch pieces

2 cups cherry tomatoes

1 15-ounce can reduced-sodium garbanzo beans,
   drained and rinsed

1 cup pitted kalamata olives

1 cup quartered artichoke hearts, drained

8 ounces fresh baby mozzarella balls, drained

1 cup packed fresh basil leaves

1 garlic clove

3 tablespoons pine nuts

⅓ cup grated Parmesan cheese

Grated zest of ½ lemon

¼ teaspoon sea salt

¼ teaspoon freshly ground black pepper

⅓ cup extra virgin olive oil

Pour an inch of water into a pot fitted with a steamer basket and bring to a simmer. Add the asparagus, cover, and steam until bright green and barely tender, 1 to 2 minutes. You want it to be crisp. Transfer the asparagus to a large bowl. Put the broccoli in the pot and steam like the asparagus. Add to the large bowl along with the cherry tomatoes, garbanzo beans, olives, artichoke hearts, and mozzarella balls.

Place the basil leaves, garlic, pine nuts, Parmesan cheese, lemon zest, salt, and pepper in a blender or food processor. Add the olive oil and pulse until the mixture forms a thick puree. Pour over the vegetables and gently toss to coat.

Tuna and White Bean Salad Open-Faced Sandwiches

Prep: 20 minutes • Cook: 0 minutes
Yield: 2 cups tuna salad; 6 sandwiches

1 15-ounce can reduced-sodium Great Northern, navy, or
   cannellini beans, drained and rinsed

2 5-ounce cans chunk light or chunk white albacore tuna in
   water, drained

1 celery rib, cut into ¼-inch dice

1 tablespoon finely chopped shallot

1 handful flat-leaf parsley, finely chopped

¼ cup finely chopped dill pickles

1 tablespoon reduced-fat olive oil mayonnaise

1 tablespoon extra virgin olive oil

1 tablespoon white wine vinegar

¼ teaspoon sea salt

½ teaspoon freshly ground black pepper

Bibb or Boston lettuce leaves, or green or red leaf lettuce

6 slices whole-grain bread, toasted, if desired

1 bunch radishes, thinly sliced

3 hard-boiled eggs, thinly sliced

Put the beans in a bowl and coarsely mash with a fork. Add the tuna, celery, shallot, parsley, pickles, mayonnaise, olive oil, vinegar, salt, and pepper. Mix thoroughly.

To assemble the sandwiches, place a lettuce leaf on each slice of bread, add ⅓ cup salad, and top with slices of radish and half a hard-boiled egg. The salad can also be eaten on a bed of mixed greens, instead of as a sandwich.

Sides

Sides can be accompaniments to meals or stand-alone lunches (or breakfasts!). Just make sure that you choose food that is not too carb heavy—you need that fiber and lean protein to keep your body and brain humming!

Jojo Potatoes

Prep: 15 minutes   •   Cook: 20 minutes
Yield: 8 servings

3 pounds russet potatoes, unpeeled, scrubbed well
2 tablespoons extra virgin olive oil
½ teaspoon finely chopped fresh thyme or rosemary,
    or ¼ teaspoon dried
½ teaspoon chili powder
¼ teaspoon garlic powder
¼ teaspoon onion powder
¼ teaspoon paprika
⅛ teaspoon celery seed
½ teaspoon sea salt
½ teaspoon freshly ground black pepper

Preheat the oven to 425°F.

Cut the potatoes in half lengthwise, then cut lengthwise into wedges 1 inch thick. Place the potato wedges in a large bowl, drizzle with the olive oil, and add the remaining ingredients. Toss to coat with the seasonings, then spread out on a baking sheet in a single layer, peel side down. Roast until golden brown and tender, about 20 minutes.

Cooking Tip: It's best to use garlic powder instead of garlic salt, because that allows you to control the amount of salt and use better-quality salt, such as unrefined sea salt. But if you do use garlic, onion, and/or celery salt, then omit the sea salt listed in the recipe so the potatoes won't be too salty.

Curry Roasted Cauliflower

Prep: 10 minutes   •   Cook: 15 to 20 minutes
Yield: five 1-cup servings

1 head cauliflower
2 tablespoons extra virgin olive oil
½ teaspoon curry powder
¼ teaspoon ground cumin
¼ teaspoon onion powder
¼ teaspoon garlic powder
½ teaspoon sea salt
½ teaspoon freshly ground black pepper
1 teaspoon lemon juice
2 tablespoons chopped fresh cilantro

Preheat the oven to 475°F.

Cut the cauliflower florets into 2-inch pieces. On a large baking sheet, combine the cauliflower, olive oil, curry powder, cumin, onion powder, garlic powder, salt, and pepper. Toss to coat and spread out in a single layer. Roast until tender and nicely browned, 15 to 20 minutes. Remove from the oven, sprinkle with lemon juice and cilantro, and serve.

Roasted Garlic Mashed Potatoes

Prep: 5 minutes • Cook: 1 hour 15 minutes
Yield: 5½ cups; about ten ½-cup servings

Cooking Tip: You can roast the garlic ahead of time; then your mashed potatoes will take only about 15 minutes to make. Just pop the roasted cloves out of their skins and add them along with the butter.

1 head garlic
1 teaspoon extra virgin olive oil
3 pounds russet potatoes, peeled and cut into 1-inch pieces
1 tablespoon organic unsalted butter
½ cup whole milk (or step up to
    2% reduced-fat milk), heated
1 teaspoon sea salt
Pinch of freshly ground white or black pepper

Preheat the oven to 375°F. Peel off the outer layers of garlic skin. Cut the garlic in half and place on a square of foil. Drizzle the cut sides with the olive oil, then put them back together. Bring the foil up around the garlic head, crimping at the top to close. Place in a pie tin or on a baking sheet, and roast until very soft and lightly browned, about 1 hour 15 minutes. Remove from the oven and open the foil to cool until comfortable to handle.

Meanwhile, add the cut potatoes to a pot filled with cold water to cover by 1 inch. Place on the stove over high heat and bring to a boil. Season with a pinch of salt. Cook the potatoes until knife tender, about 10 minutes. Drain the potatoes and place them back in the pot. Return the pot to the stove to keep warm over low heat. Using a potato masher or sturdy balloon whisk, mash the potatoes thoroughly. Add the butter and squeeze the roasted garlic out of its skin into the potatoes. Stir to combine. Stir in half of the heated milk. If the potatoes are too thick, stir in the remaining milk. Season with salt and pepper, stirring to combine.

Turkey and Brown Rice Patties

Prep: 10 minutes   •   Cook: 8 minutes
Yield: 6 patties

Cooking Tip: These patties are a great jumping-off point from which you can get creative with the flavorings. Try different herbs such as tarragon, oregano, or rosemary. You can change up the spices by using curry powder, Cajun seasonings, or Italian herb and spice blends. Just make sure they're salt-free!

Try adding one of these patties to the Fast-Food Lunch
(page 190) for a complete meal!

½ pound lean ground turkey
2 cups cooked brown rice (leftover is fine, or use any cooked
    whole grain, such as quinoa, barley, or bulgur)
¼ cup dried whole-wheat bread crumbs
1 tablespoon ketchup
1 tablespoon Dijon mustard
1 small handful of basil, parsley, or cilantro,
    chopped
¼ teaspoon garlic powder
¼ teaspoon onion powder
¼ teaspoon paprika (regular, smoked, or sweet)
¼ teaspoon ground cumin
½ teaspoon sea salt
¼ teaspoon freshly ground black pepper
1 teaspoon extra virgin olive oil (or step up to
    Eat-Clean cooking spray)

In a large bowl, combine all of the ingredients, except for the olive oil. Mix together until combined thoroughly.

Divide the mixture into 6 equal portions and shape into patties.

Heat a large nonstick skillet over medium-low heat and add the olive oil (or spray with Eat-Clean cooking spray). You want to give the patties plenty of cooking room, so you might need to cook them in two batches. Add the patties in a single layer and cook until browned and no longer pink in the center, about 4 minutes on each side. Serve immediately. These can be eaten "naked" (without a bun), "topless" (open-faced), or "traditional" on a hamburger bun—just make it whole grain!

Leftover patties will keep in the refrigerator for up to 3 days, or in the freezer for up to 3 months. They can be reheated in a 350°F oven or toaster oven.

Main Meals

These Start Here recipes are fast, delicious, and filling! Even though I most often list them in the meal plans as dinner suggestions, you can enjoy them for any meal of the day.

Hawaiian Chicken Burger

Prep: 15 minutes • Cook: 15 minutes
Yield: 4 burgers

1 pound ground chicken or turkey

2 scallions, finely chopped

2 tablespoons finely chopped fresh cilantro

1 teaspoon toasted sesame oil

¼ teaspoon sea salt

½ teaspoon freshly ground black pepper

1 20-ounce can sliced pineapple in its own juice (you will
   need 8 slices of pineapple and ½ cup pineapple juice)

1 teaspoon cornstarch or arrowroot

1 tablespoon low-sodium soy sauce

1 tablespoon honey

½ teaspoon garlic powder

1 teaspoon extra virgin olive oil

½ sweet onion, thinly sliced

Eat-Clean cooking spray

4 whole-grain hamburger buns, toasted

4 teaspoons Dijon or yellow mustard

4 teaspoons reduced-fat olive oil mayonnaise

In a bowl, combine the ground chicken, scallions, cilantro, sesame oil, salt, and pepper. Use a wooden spoon or clean hands to mix together. Form into 4 patties.

Pour ½ cup pineapple juice into a small saucepan. Add the

cornstarch or arrowroot and whisk to combine. Add the soy sauce, honey, and garlic powder. Turn the heat to medium-high and bring to a bubble, stirring as it thickens. Remove from heat and set aside.

Heat the olive oil in a nonstick pan over medium-high heat. Add the onion and cook until soft and caramelized, 5 minutes. Transfer to a plate.

Return the skillet to the stove and reduce the heat to medium low. Spray with cooking spray and add the chicken patties. Cook until no longer pink in the middle, turning once, 3 to 5 minutes on each side.

To build the burgers, spread mustard and mayonnaise on the buns, add a cooked chicken patty, 2 slices of pineapple, some sautéed onion, and drizzle with the sauce. Serve immediately.

Sloppy Joe Sandwiches

Prep: 15 minutes • Cook: 20 minutes
Yield: 6 cups; six 1-cup servings

1 15-ounce can tomato sauce

2 tablespoons tomato paste

1 tablespoon Dijon mustard

1 tablespoon molasses

1 tablespoon apple cider vinegar

1 tablespoon Worcestershire sauce

1 teaspoon Mexican-style hot sauce

1 tablespoon extra virgin olive oil

1 onion, chopped

2 celery ribs, finely chopped

1 green bell pepper, seeded and finely chopped

1 cup shredded carrot

1¼ pounds ground turkey

1 teaspoon ground cumin

1 teaspoon chili powder

½ teaspoon garlic powder

¼ teaspoon sea salt

½ teaspoon freshly ground black pepper

6 whole-grain hamburger buns, split in half

In a small bowl, whisk together the tomato sauce, tomato paste, Dijon mustard, molasses, vinegar, Worcestershire sauce, and hot sauce, and set aside.

Heat the olive oil in a very large nonstick skillet over medium-high heat. Add the onion, celery, green pepper, and carrot and cook until soft and starting to brown, 10 minutes. Push the vegetables to the side. Add the turkey and cook, breaking it up with a wooden spoon until no longer pink, 5 minutes. Add the cumin, chili powder, garlic powder, salt, and pepper, and stir in the seasonings. Add the reserved tomato sauce mixture and stir to combine. Cover and simmer for 3 minutes. Scoop onto hamburger buns (or whole-grain bread or brown rice, if you prefer).

Quinoa Black Bean Burgers

Prep: 20 minutes • Cook: 10 minutes
Yield: four 4-inch burgers

You may not yet be familiar with quinoa, or maybe you even think of it as weird because its name looks so hard to pronounce (it's easy: KEEN-wah). Have no fear! Quinoa is one of the most nutritionally complete grains (it's what nutritionists call a complete protein) and is so quick and easy to prepare I love it as a substitute for pasta. But if you are not ready to try this delicious morsel, then replace it in the recipe that follows with brown rice, bulgur, or barley.

1 15-ounce can black beans, drained and rinsed

2 cups cooked quinoa (you can also use brown rice, bulgur, or barley)

¼ cup finely chopped fresh cilantro

2 tablespoons finely chopped chives or scallions
  (green parts only)

¼ teaspoon garlic powder

¼ teaspoon ground cumin

¼ teaspoon chili powder

1 teaspoon Mexican-style hot sauce, plus more for
  the dressing, if desired

¼ cup dried whole-wheat bread crumbs

2 tablespoons grated Parmesan cheese

1 egg

½ teaspoon sea salt, plus a pinch for the dressing

¼ teaspoon freshly ground black pepper,
  plus a pinch for the dressing

1 tablespoon extra virgin olive oil

1 tablespoon reduced-fat olive oil mayonnaise

¼ cup Greek yogurt, drained

1 teaspoon fresh lime juice

4 whole-grain burger buns

Burger fixings, such as lettuce, tomato, and sliced onion

Place the black beans in a large bowl and mash well with a fork. Add the quinoa, cilantro, chives, garlic powder, cumin, chili powder, hot sauce, bread crumbs, Parmesan, egg, salt, and pepper.

Mix the ingredients together thoroughly for a few minutes with a wooden spoon or your hands. Form a patty to test the consistency. The mixture should hold its shape easily and be moist, but not too sticky. If it's too moist, then add a few more dried bread crumbs. If it's too dry, add a tablespoon or two of milk.

Divide the mixture into 4 equal portions and shape into patties.

Heat the olive oil in a large nonstick skillet over medium heat. Add the patties in a single layer and cook until browned and heated through, about 5 minutes on each side.

Meanwhile, in a small bowl, mix together the mayonnaise, yogurt, lime juice, and hot sauce, if using, and season with a pinch of salt and pepper.

To build your burger, spread the lime-yogurt mixture on the bun, add a quinoa black bean patty, and top with your favorite burger fixings.

Italian Ragu over Pasta

Prep: 10 minutes • Cook: 40 minutes
Yield: six 1-cup servings

Ragu is an Italian sauce that is traditionally served with pasta. But it's also delicious over whole grains such as brown rice (or quinoa!) and steamed or grilled vegetables.

½ yellow or white onion, cut into large chunks

1 carrot, peeled and cut into large chunks

1 celery rib, cut into large chunks

2 cups white button or cremini mushrooms

2 garlic cloves

2 tablespoons extra virgin olive oil

1 pound lean ground beef (or step up to lean ground turkey, or a combination)

½ teaspoon salt

½ teaspoon black pepper

1 teaspoon dried oregano or dried Italian herbs

1 tablespoon tomato paste

½ cup dry red wine

1 28-ounce can crushed tomatoes (preferably low-salt or no-salt)

1 cup whole milk (or step up to reduced-fat milk)

Whole-grain spaghetti, linguini, fettuccini, or similar pasta

Fresh basil leaves, thinly sliced, to garnish

In a food processor, pulse the onion, carrot, celery, mushrooms, and garlic until finely chopped, or finely chop with a large knife.

Heat the olive oil in a large pot over medium-high heat. Add the chopped vegetables and cook, stirring occasionally, until softened, about 5 minutes. Add the beef or turkey, salt, pepper, and oregano, breaking up the meat with a wooden spoon, and cook until no longer pink, about 5 minutes. Add the tomato paste, red wine, tomatoes, and milk. Bring to a boil, then reduce the heat and simmer, partially covered, until slightly thickened, about 30 minutes. Stir occasionally to prevent the bottom from sticking.

When the ragu is almost done, bring a large pot of salted water to a boil and cook the pasta according to package directions. Drain the pasta and toss with the ragu. To serve, mound in bowls and top with fresh basil.

Cooking Tip: This ragu makes great leftovers! It can be refrigerated for up to 5 days or frozen for up to 3 months.

Peanut Noodles with Chicken and Vegetables

Prep: 15 minutes   •   Cook: 15 minutes
Yield: 10 cups; five 2-cup servings

1 teaspoon extra virgin olive oil

1 pound boneless, skinless chicken breasts or thighs

¼ teaspoon sea salt

¼ teaspoon freshly ground black pepper

8 ounces whole-wheat linguini, spaghetti,
   or similar long pasta

½ cup natural peanut butter, at room temperature

¼ cup rice vinegar or apple cider vinegar

¼ cup warm water

2 tablespoons low-sodium soy sauce

2 tablespoons honey

½ teaspoon red pepper flakes, or more to taste

2 cups shredded carrots

2 cups bite-size broccoli florets

2 scallions, finely chopped

1 red or yellow bell pepper, seeded and thinly sliced
   into 1-inch strips

1 tablespoon sesame seeds

Preheat the oven to 400°F. Heat the olive oil in an ovenproof skillet over medium-high heat. Season the chicken with salt and pepper and add it to the pan in a single layer. Cook until golden brown on one side, turn over, and place in the preheated oven to finish cooking, about 7 minutes. To test doneness, cut one breast open. If it's no longer pink in the thickest part and the juices run clear, it's ready. Remove from the oven and let rest for a few minutes.

Meanwhile, bring a large pot of salted water to boil over high heat. Add the pasta and cook according to package directions until tender, but firm to the bite. Drain and place in a large bowl.

In a small bowl, whisk together the peanut butter, vinegar, water, soy sauce, honey, and red pepper flakes, and pour over the pasta. Add the carrots, broccoli, scallions, bell pepper, and sesame seeds. Dice the cooked chicken and add to the bowl.

Toss to combine, coating all the ingredients with the peanut sauce. The dish can be served immediately or made ahead of time and refrigerated for up to 3 days.

Tip: If you want more heat in your peanut noodles, top them with Asian chili sauce.

Pepper Pot Soup

This is a classic Jamaican dish that everyone on the island grows up eating, and every Jamaican mom has her own version. This healthy, hearty rendition has some spicy heat—and it's the kind that creeps up on you. If you are sensitive to spicy food, either remove the chile pepper after 15 minutes of cooking, or omit it entirely.

Prep: 15 minutes • Cook: 2½ hours
Yield: 13 cups; thirteen 1-cup servings

1 pound beef stew meat, trimmed of excess fat and
    cut into 1-inch pieces (to make your life easier,
    look for stew meat already cubed)
2 celery ribs, cut into ½-inch dice
2 large carrots, peeled and cut into ½-inch dice
2 quarts low-sodium chicken broth
1 quart water
1 pound collard greens, stalks removed,
    finely chopped
1 russet potato, peeled and cut into ½-inch dice
1 sweet potato, peeled and cut into ½-inch dice
3 scallions, chopped
1 cup sliced okra (frozen or fresh)
1 Scotch bonnet pepper or habañero chile,
    stemmed but whole
3 garlic cloves, finely chopped
1 tablespoon chopped fresh thyme, or 1 teaspoon dried
1 teaspoon sea salt
1 teaspoon freshly ground black pepper
½ cup unsweetened canned coconut milk

Put the beef, celery, and carrots in a large pot or Dutch oven, cover with chicken broth and water, and bring to a boil over high heat. Reduce to a simmer, cover, and cook for 2 hours. Uncover and add the collard greens, potato, sweet potato, scallions, okra, Scotch bonnet pepper, garlic, thyme, salt, and black pepper. Bring to a boil over high heat, then reduce to a simmer and cook, covered, for 30 minutes, until the beef and vegetables are very tender. Remove the Scotch bonnet pepper and discard. Stir in the coconut milk. Ladle into bowls and serve.

Spicy Shrimp and Sausage Gumbo

Prep: 20 minutes • Cook: 30 minutes
Yield: 10 cups; ten 1-cup servings of gumbo
with ½ cup brown rice

4 tablespoons olive oil
¼ cup whole-wheat flour
1 onion, diced small
2 celery ribs, diced small
1 green pepper, diced small
3 garlic cloves, minced
1 teaspoon sea salt
½ teaspoon freshly ground black pepper
½ teaspoon Old Bay seasoning
¼ teaspoon cayenne (or ½ teaspoon for a very spicy gumbo)
¼ teaspoon poultry seasoning (salt free)
1 quart low-sodium chicken broth
2 cups frozen sliced okra
1 15-ounce can diced tomatoes, drained
2 tablespoons tomato paste
1 tablespoon Worcestershire sauce
1 pound large raw shrimp, peeled and deveined
14 ounces low-fat all natural fully cooked sausage, such as
    andouille or kielbasa, cut into ½-inch rounds
5 cups cooked brown rice
½ cup finely chopped scallions (green part only)
Hot pepper sauce

Heat 3 tablespoons of the olive oil in a small heavy saucepan over medium heat. Add the flour and whisk regularly until it has the aroma of popcorn, 3 minutes. Remove from heat and set aside.

In a large soup pot or Dutch oven, heat the remaining 1 tablespoon olive oil over moderate heat. Add the onion and cook until soft and translucent, 5 minutes. Add the celery, green pepper, and garlic and cook for 5 minutes, until tender, stirring occasion-ally. Season with the salt, black pepper, Old Bay, cayenne, and poultry seasoning.

Add the reserved cooked flour mixture and stir until all the vegetables are coated. Slowly whisk in the chicken broth. Add the okra, tomatoes, tomato paste, and Worcestershire sauce. Stir to combine.

Bring to a boil over high heat, then reduce the heat and sim-mer for 15 minutes. Increase the heat to a gentle boil. Gently stir in the shrimp and sausage. Simmer for 3 more minutes, until the shrimp are cooked through.

Portion the rice into bowls, top with gumbo, and garnish with scallions. Serve with hot pepper sauce.

Lemon and Herb Crusted Cod

Prep: 10 minutes   •   Cook: 10 to 12 minutes
Yield: 4 servings

Eat-Clean cooking spray
⅔ cup dried whole-wheat bread crumbs (You can use crushed
   almonds instead of the bread crumbs to step it up)
Grated zest of 1 large lemon
1 tablespoon finely chopped parsley, dill, or basil
2 tablespoons grated Parmesan cheese
½ teaspoon garlic powder
½ teaspoon sea salt
¼ teaspoon freshly ground black pepper
⅛ teaspoon white pepper
1 egg
2 tablespoons milk
4 cod fillets, 4 to 6 ounces each
Lemon wedges

Preheat the oven to 450°F. Coat a baking sheet with Eat-Clean cooking spray.

In a shallow dish, stir together the bread crumbs, lemon zest, parsley, Parmesan, garlic powder, salt, black pepper, and white pepper.

In a separate shallow dish, beat together the egg and milk. Dip the cod in the egg mixture, turning to coat, then place in the bread crumb or almond mixture. Press the crumbs onto one side of the cod to lightly coat, then turn and press onto the other side. Gently shake to remove excess crumbs; place on the baking sheet. Bake 10 to 12 minutes, until the cod gently flakes with a fork. Serve with lemon wedges.

One-Skillet Sweet and Sour Chicken

Prep: 10 minutes   •   Cook: 15 minutes

Yield: four 2-cup servings

¼ cup honey

¼ cup white vinegar

1 tablespoon reduced-sodium soy sauce

1 teaspoon tomato paste

1 tablespoon cornstarch (or arrowroot)

½ teaspoon sea salt

1 tablespoon extra virgin olive oil

1 pound boneless, skinless chicken breasts, cut
    into 1-inch dice

½ red onion, cut into 1-inch dice

¼ teaspoon freshly ground black pepper

4 cups frozen stir-fry vegetables

1 8-ounce can pineapple chunks in juice, undrained

1 cup water

2 cups instant or quick-cooking whole-grain brown rice
    (parcooked whole-grain brown rice that cooks
    in 10 minutes or less)

In a bowl, whisk together the honey, vinegar, soy sauce, tomato paste, cornstarch, and ¼ teaspoon of the sea salt. Set aside.

Heat the olive oil in a large skillet over medium-high heat. Add the chicken and onion, and season with pepper and the remaining ¼ teaspoon salt. Cook, stirring occasionally, for 5 minutes.

Add the vegetables, pineapple chunks and their juice, and the reserved sauce mixture. Stir in the water and bring to a boil.

Stir in the rice and cover. Reduce the heat to medium low and simmer for 5 minutes. Remove from heat and let stand, covered, for 5 minutes. Uncover and serve.

Taco Night

Prep: 15 minutes   •   Cook: 10 minutes
Yield: 4½ cups; makes about 8 soft tacos

8 8-inch whole-grain soft taco-size tortillas (or step up to sprouted whole-grain tortillas, such as Ezekiel)

Taco Fillings:
1 teaspoon extra virgin olive oil
½ onion, finely chopped
1½ pounds lean or extra-lean ground beef (or step up to lean ground turkey or chicken, or a combination)
1 teaspoon Mexican chili powder
1 teaspoon ground cumin
1 teaspoon garlic powder
¼ teaspoon sea salt
½ teaspoon freshly ground black pepper
1 16-ounce can fat-free or low-fat refried beans

Taco Fixings:
Shredded romaine lettuce
Chopped tomatoes
Chopped red onion or scallions
Chopped avocado

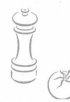

Chopped fresh cilantro
Greek yogurt
Mexican hot sauce

Heat the olive oil in a very large nonstick skillet over moderate heat. Add the onion and cook until soft, about 5 minutes. Increase the heat to medium high and add the ground beef (or turkey or chicken); use a wooden spoon to break it up as it cooks. Stir in the chili powder, cumin, garlic powder, salt, and pepper. Continue to cook the beef until it is no longer pink. Stir in the beans.

Serve on whole-grain tortillas with your favorite taco fixings, such as lettuce, tomatoes, and avocado. Top with a little hot sauce, if desired.

Whole Roasted Chicken with Natural Pan Gravy

Prep: 15 minutes   •   Cook: 1 to 1½ hours
Yield: Chicken—4 to 6 servings; gravy—1½ cups

Roasted Chicken:
1 4- to 5-pound chicken
1 lemon, quartered
1 teaspoon extra virgin olive oil
½ teaspoon sea salt
¼ teaspoon black pepper

½ teaspoon poultry seasoning (**or** ½ teaspoon combination of your favorite dried herbs and spices, such as thyme, marjoram, sage, rosemary, paprika, cumin, coriander, or nutmeg; **or** 1 teaspoon of your favorite fresh herbs, minced, such as rosemary, thyme, or sage)

Gravy:
Drippings from the roasted chicken
1¼ cups low-sodium chicken broth

1 tablespoon cornstarch or arrowroot

Juice from the lemons inside the roasted chicken

Pinch of sea salt and freshly ground black pepper

To make the chicken:

Preheat the oven to 375°F.

Remove the packet from inside the chicken (containing the neck and innards) and either discard or save for future use (the neck can be used to make stock; the liver can be used to make paté). Rinse the chicken inside and out with cold water, drain, and pat dry with a paper towel.

Place the chicken on a shallow roasting pan or baking sheet with a lip, breast side up. The legs will be angled up and the wings will be on the bottom. Tuck the wings underneath the body to keep them from burning.

Place the lemon quarters inside the chicken.

Rub the outside of the chicken thoroughly with the olive oil, wipe off your hands, and season the chicken all over with salt, pepper, and the herbs/spices of your choice. Pat or gently rub the seasonings into the skin. Wash your hands.

Roast the chicken until browned and the internal temperature reaches 165 degrees. A 5-pound chicken will take about 1½ hours to cook. If you don't have a thermometer, you can check by making a cut near the leg; if the juices run clear, the chicken is done.

Remove the chicken from the oven. Remove the lemons with tongs or a fork and set aside. Cover the chicken with foil and let it rest for 10 minutes.

To make the gravy:

Spoon off and discard the fat that floated to the top of the drippings in the roasting pan. Pour the remaining liquid into a small pan and place on the stove over medium-high heat.

Add 1 cup of the chicken broth and bring to a simmer.

In a small bowl, whisk together the remaining ¼ cup chicken broth with the cornstarch or arrowroot and add to the pot while whisking constantly.

Simmer the gravy until it thickens, about 1 minute.

Remove from heat, squeeze in the juice from the lemon quarters you set aside, and season with salt and pepper.

To serve, carve the chicken and serve with the natural pan gravy.

Corned Beef with Cabbage, Potatoes, and Root Vegetables

Prep: 15 minutes   •   Cook: 3 hours
Yield: 6 to 8 servings

Corned Beef:

1 3- to 4-pound uncooked corned beef brisket, in brine

2 tablespoons whole-grain Dijon mustard

1 tablespoon honey

Horseradish Sauce:

1 cup Greek yogurt, drained

2 tablespoons jarred grated horseradish, with liquid

½ teaspoon finely grated lemon zest

¼ teaspoon sea salt

¼ teaspoon freshly ground black pepper, or more to taste

Potatoes and Root Vegetables:

1 pound small yellow or red potatoes, halved

2 large carrots, peeled and cut into 1-inch pieces

2 large parsnips, peeled and cut into 1-inch pieces

1 large or two smaller turnips or rutabagas, peeled and cut into 1-inch pieces

Cabbage:

1 tablespoon extra virgin olive oil

1 medium yellow onion, halved and thinly sliced

½ large head green cabbage, cored and thinly sliced

1 garlic clove, finely chopped

½ teaspoon freshly ground black pepper

2 tablespoons of the reserved roasted
   corned beef cooking liquid

To make the corned beef:

Preheat the oven to 350°F.

Remove the corned beef from the packing and set the spice packet aside. Place the corned beef in a colander in the sink and rinse under cold running water. To extract the extra salt, place the corned beef in a large pot and cover with cold water. Bring to a boil over high heat for 1 minute, then discard the water. Repeat with more fresh water, boiling for 1 minute, then discarding the water again. Transfer the beef to a shallow roasting pan or baking dish just big enough to hold the meat, fat side up.

In a small bowl, mix together the mustard and honey and spread three fourths of it across the top and sides of the corned beef. Cover the dish with a fitted lid or foil, making sure there's space between the lid or foil and the top of the beef. Roast for 2 to 3 hours, until the meat is cooked through and you can easily pull it apart with a fork. Uncover the corned beef, spread the rest of the honey-mustard mixture over the top, and place under the broiler until lightly browned, 2 minutes. Scoop out 2 tablespoons of the liquid from the bottom of the roasting pan and set aside. Allow the beef to rest for 10 minutes.

To make the horseradish sauce:

Meanwhile, in a small bowl, mix together the yogurt, horseradish, lemon zest, salt, and pepper and refrigerate until ready to serve. The sauce can be made a day ahead.

To make the potatoes and root vegetables:

Bring a large pot of water to a boil over high heat. Place the ingredients of the spice packet in a tea strainer (or in the middle of two layers of cheesecloth, shaped into a small bundle and tied with a piece of butcher's string) and add to the water. Add the potatoes, carrots, parsnips, and turnips. Simmer until the potatoes and vegetables are tender, about 15 minutes. Drain. Cover to keep warm until ready to serve.

To make the cabbage:

Heat the olive oil in a very large skillet or Dutch oven over medium heat. Add the onion and cook until soft and starting to brown. Add the cabbage, garlic, and pepper, and stir to combine. Continue to cook until the cabbage is soft and starting to brown. Add the reserved roasted corned beef cooking liquid, stir it into the cabbage, and cook until evaporated.

To serve, slice the corned beef across the grain. Serve with the boiled potatoes and root vegetables, cabbage, and horseradish sauce.

Mandarin Shrimp Salad

Prep: 20 minutes • Cook: 0 minutes
Yield: 12 cups; four 3-cup main course servings;
eight 1½-cup side dish servings

This salad is so easy to make because there's no cooking required! Simply thaw the shrimp if using frozen shrimp, let them marinate for a little bit in the fridge while you assemble the rest of the ingredients, then toss everything together and you're ready to eat!

Tip: If you can't find Mandarin oranges, use navel oranges.

1 pound large cooked shrimp, peeled, deveined, tails
   removed, and chopped into bite-size pieces
   (if using frozen, thaw first)
3 Mandarin oranges, 1 juiced; 2 peeled, segmented,
   and cut into bite-size pieces
1 red bell pepper, seeded and thinly sliced into
   bite-size pieces
2 tablespoons grapeseed oil
1 teaspoon toasted sesame oil

1 tablespoon fresh lime juice

½ teaspoon sea salt

½ teaspoon freshly ground black pepper

4 cups thinly sliced green cabbage

4 cups thinly sliced romaine lettuce

2 scallions, finely chopped

¼ cup chopped fresh cilantro

½ cup sliced almonds

In a large bowl, combine the shrimp, Mandarin orange juice and segments, bell pepper, grapeseed oil, sesame oil, lime juice, salt, and pepper. Mix together and refrigerate for 15 minutes, or up to 1 hour.

In a large salad bowl, combine the cabbage, lettuce, scallions, and cilantro.

Toast the almonds in a pan over moderate heat until golden, stirring frequently, about 5 minutes. Add to the salad bowl.

Add the refrigerated shrimp mixture to the salad. Toss to combine and serve.

Desserts

I consider dessert a treat, an indulgence, and a necessity—every now and then! The key to enjoying dessert is to partake in moderation, which is why you don't even see desserts in my meal plans. I trust you understand that too much of a sweet good thing will end up making you just feel bad all over.

Chocolate-Chocolate Chip Zucchini Cake

Prep: 20 minutes • Cook: 50 minutes
Yield: 16 servings

Eat-Clean cooking spray, for preparing the pan
All-purpose flour, for preparing the pan

Wet Ingredients:
2 eggs
1 cup buttermilk
½ cup unsweetened applesauce
½ cup coconut oil, softened
½ cup packed brown sugar
1 teaspoon vanilla extract

Dry Ingredients:
1½ cups whole-wheat flour
1 cup all-purpose flour
¼ cup unsweetened cocoa powder
1 teaspoon baking soda
½ teaspoon cinnamon
¼ teaspoon ground cloves
¼ teaspoon sea salt

2 cups grated zucchini

¼ cup chopped walnuts (optional)

¼ cup semisweet chocolate chips (optional)

Preheat the oven to 325°F. Grease and flour a 9 x 9-inch baking pan.

In a large bowl, whisk together the wet ingredients until thoroughly combined. In a separate bowl, sift the dry ingredients. Add the dry ingredients to the wet ingredients and stir together until just combined. Stir in the grated zucchini.

Scrape the batter into the prepared pan and smooth out the surface. Top with the chocolate chips and chopped walnuts, if desired.

Bake for 50 to 55 minutes, until a toothpick inserted into the center comes out clean. Allow to sit at room temperature for 10 minutes, then cut and serve.

Mini Cherry Berry Pies

Cherry pie is an American classic. But the kind you find in the grocery store is usually made with shortening that contains hydrogenated fat (not good for you), plus a lot of sugar as well as red food coloring. These mini pies are cleaned up so that they're more healthful, and they have berries, too! They're also very easy to make because there's no lattice crust to fuss with. In fact, you don't even use a pie dish!

Cooking Tip: You can "step up" to using all whole-wheat flour; just add 1 tablespoon of water when making the dough to ensure that it is moist enough.

Prep: 25 minutes active, 20 minutes inactive   •   Cook: 40 minutes
Yield: 6 mini pies

Crust:

½ cup all-purpose flour, plus more for rolling the dough

½ cup whole-wheat flour

¼ teaspoon sea salt

6 tablespoons coconut oil, chilled

¼ cup ice water

Filling:

2 cups pitted frozen pie cherries, thawed slightly

1 cup frozen raspberries, blackberries, or
     sliced strawberries, thawed slightly

⅓ cup packed brown sugar

2 tablespoons apple or orange juice, or water

1 tablespoon cornstarch or arrowroot

1 teaspoon almond extract

Pinch of sea salt

Topping:

1 teaspoon brown sugar

⅛ teaspoon cinnamon

⅛ teaspoon nutmeg

1 tablespoon milk

Preheat the oven to 375°F. Place 6 3-oz. ramekins on a baking sheet.

To make the crust, sift the flours and salt into a bowl. Cut in the coconut oil until crumbly. Gradually add the water a little at a time, stirring with a fork until the dough starts to come together. The pie crust can be made in a food processor to make it even easier. Gather the dough into a ball; shape into a disk. Wrap in plastic and refrigerate for 20 minutes.

In a large bowl, mix the cherries, berries, brown sugar, juice or water, cornstarch, almond extract, and salt. Divide the fruit mixture among the ramekins.

Dust a large, flat work surface with a little flour. Remove the dough from the fridge, unwrap, and place on the surface. Dust a rolling pin with a little flour and roll out the dough into a 9-inch disk. Use a round cookie cutter about the same size as the ramekins to cut 6 mini crusts, and place them on the cherry berry mixture.

For the topping, combine the brown sugar with the cinnamon

and nutmeg. Brush the crusts with milk and sprinkle the top of each pie with the sugar and spices.

Place on the middle rack of the oven and bake until golden brown and bubbling, about 40 minutes.

Ricotta and Blackberry Crepes

If you're intimidated by crepes, don't be! They're basically thin pancakes stuffed with a tasty filling. For this dessert I use blackberries, but you could also use strawberries, blueberries, or raspberries. This dessert is easy to make, and it's one the whole family will love! It's also an impressive finale for a dinner party. The berries and ricotta can be prepared ahead of time, and even the crepes can be cooked a day ahead, so when it's time for dessert, simply assemble and enjoy!

Prep: 30 minutes • Cook: 10 minutes
Yield: 4 crepes

Crepe Batter:

½ cup low-fat milk
½ cup water
1 cup whole-wheat flour
2 eggs
1 tablespoon coconut oil, melted
Pinch of sea salt

Crepe Filling:

2 cups frozen blackberries
2 tablespoons plus 1 teaspoon honey
2 teaspoons cornstarch or arrowroot
¼ teaspoon cinnamon
1 cup reduced-fat (or light, or low-fat) ricotta cheese
¼ teaspoon vanilla extract
1 teaspoon finely grated lemon zest

Eat-Clean cooking spray

Combine all crepe batter ingredients in a blender. Blend until smooth and free of lumps. You can also whisk the ingredients together in a bowl. Refrigerate the batter for 10 minutes.

Meanwhile, in a small saucepan, combine the blackberries, the 2 tablespoons honey, the cornstarch, and cinnamon. Bring to a bubble over medium-high heat, stirring until thickened. Set aside to cool to room temperature.

In a small bowl, mix the ricotta cheese, vanilla extract, lemon zest, and remaining 1 teaspoon honey.

Heat a 10-inch nonstick skillet over medium heat and lightly coat with Eat-Clean cooking spray. Pour ⅓ cup of crepe batter into the pan and swirl to coat the bottom. Let the batter cook until it sets up, 30 to 60 seconds. Using a rubber spatula, loosen the edges and flip the crepe. Cook for another 10 seconds, then slide it out onto a plate. The crepe should be golden brown and tender. Repeat until all the batter is used. There should be enough batter for 5 crepes, allowing one for practice or extra nibbles.

To assemble, spread ¼ cup of the cheese filling down one side of each crepe. Spread ¼ cup blackberry mixture down the other side. Fold the two sides together, and fold in half again. Serve immediately.

Tip: This is a great dessert to make year round because it uses frozen berries. If fresh berries are in season, or other fresh tender fruits such as apricots, plums, or peaches are available, then you don't have to cook the fruit. Just cut it into bite-size pieces, if necessary, and mix with the other filling ingredients.

Tropical Shake

Chase away your winter blues with this delicious and easy taste of the tropics. You can find frozen tropical fruit in the freezer section of your grocery.

Preparation Tip: Very ripe bananas (even bananas that have turned dark brown!) are a great way to sweeten shakes and smoothies (and other desserts, too) without using refined sugar. Once they start to turn brown, they can be stored in the refrigerator. You can also peel them and freeze them in resealable plastic bags.

TNT:

✳ You can enjoy this tropical shake for breakfast or a quick lunch; just add a tablespoon of protein powder and you're all set!

Prep: 5 minutes • Cook: 0 minutes

Yield: four 1-cup servings

1 cup plain low-fat yogurt

1 cup frozen cut tropical fruit, such as pineapple and
    mangoes (or any other frozen fruit you like,
    such as strawberries, grapes, or raspberries)

½ very ripe banana (it can even be brown)

½ cup pineapple juice

½ cup unsweetened canned coconut milk

1 tablespoon fresh lime juice

1 cup ice cubes

Shredded, unsweetened coconut,
    to garnish (optional)

Put all of the ingredients except the shredded coconut in a blender and blend until smooth. Pour into glasses and top with a little shredded coconut, if desired. Serve immediately.

Tip: Pour the shake into popsicle molds and freeze for a tropical frozen treat!

Some Final Thoughts

Life is a journey. It will always have its challenges and its possibilities. While I was writing this book, my husband, Robert, was diagnosed with a rare disease and died quite precipitously. I lost a lot—my best friend, my mentor, my inspiration, and my partner. But even as I grieved, and I grieve still, I realize that yet again he has brought me a lesson. This time my lesson is about truly embracing the difficult times in our lives and looking for how to move through them, and how to give back to the world through one's gifts and strengths.

I have designed my Start Here plan with loving care. It embodies all that I hope for, all that I wish for my daughters, and all that I continue to aspire to be. In one word, this book embodies health, which I know will lead to happiness.

As the French say, *bon courage* and *bon voyage*—wishing you lots of courage and a safe and happy journey, my friends, and hope to see you visiting our site!

Resources

_____

Your Medical Numbers

It's important to know what levels you are shooting for when it comes to blood pressure and cholesterol. Maintaining blood pressure and cholesterol at these healthy levels can lower your risk for disease and help keep your disease under control if you've already been diagnosed.

Healthy levels of cholesterol are:

> LDL levels less than 100 mg/dl
> HDL levels 60 mg/dl or higher
> Triglycerides under 150 mg/dl

A healthy blood pressure reading is 130/80 or lower.
See your doctor regularly and follow her advice.

The Body Mass Index

Body Mass Index Table

Height (inches)	Normal						Overweight					Obese										Extreme Obesity														
BMI	19	20	21	22	23	24	25	26	27	28	29	30	31	32	33	34	35	36	37	38	39	40	41	42	43	44	45	46	47	48	49	50	51	52	53	54
												Body Weight (pounds)																								
58	91	96	100	105	110	115	119	124	129	134	138	143	148	153	158	162	167	172	177	181	186	191	196	201	205	210	215	220	224	229	234	239	244	248	253	258
59	94	99	104	109	114	119	124	128	133	138	143	148	153	158	163	168	173	178	183	188	193	198	203	208	212	217	222	227	232	237	242	247	252	257	262	267
60	97	102	107	112	118	123	128	133	138	143	148	153	158	163	168	174	179	184	189	194	199	204	209	215	220	225	230	235	240	245	250	255	261	266	271	276
61	100	106	111	116	122	127	132	137	143	148	153	158	164	169	174	180	185	190	195	201	206	211	217	222	227	232	238	243	248	254	259	264	269	275	280	285
62	104	109	115	120	126	131	136	142	147	153	158	164	169	175	180	186	191	196	202	207	213	218	224	229	235	240	246	251	256	262	267	273	278	284	289	295
63	107	113	118	124	130	135	141	146	152	158	163	169	175	180	186	191	197	203	208	214	220	225	231	237	242	248	254	259	265	270	278	282	287	293	299	304
64	110	116	122	128	134	140	145	151	157	163	169	174	180	186	192	197	204	209	215	221	227	232	238	244	250	256	262	267	273	279	285	291	296	302	308	314
65	114	120	126	132	138	144	150	156	162	168	174	180	186	192	198	204	210	216	222	228	234	240	246	252	258	264	270	276	282	288	294	300	306	312	318	324
66	118	124	130	136	142	148	155	161	167	173	179	186	192	198	204	210	216	223	229	235	241	247	253	260	266	272	278	284	291	297	303	309	315	322	328	334
67	121	127	134	140	146	153	159	166	172	178	185	191	198	204	211	217	223	230	236	242	249	255	261	268	274	280	287	293	299	306	312	319	325	331	338	344
68	125	131	138	144	151	158	164	171	177	184	190	197	203	210	216	223	230	236	243	249	256	262	269	276	282	289	295	302	308	315	322	328	335	341	348	354
69	128	135	142	149	155	162	169	176	182	189	196	203	209	216	223	230	236	243	250	257	263	270	277	284	291	297	304	311	318	324	331	338	345	351	358	365
70	132	139	146	153	160	167	174	181	188	195	202	209	216	222	229	236	243	250	257	264	271	278	285	292	299	306	313	320	327	334	341	348	355	362	369	376
71	136	143	150	157	165	172	179	186	193	200	208	215	222	229	236	243	250	257	265	272	279	286	293	301	308	315	322	329	338	343	351	358	365	372	379	386
72	140	147	154	162	169	177	184	191	199	206	213	221	228	235	242	250	258	265	272	279	287	294	302	309	316	324	331	338	346	353	361	368	375	383	390	397
73	144	151	159	166	174	182	189	197	204	212	219	227	235	242	250	257	265	272	280	288	295	302	310	318	325	333	340	348	355	363	371	378	386	393	401	408
74	148	155	163	171	179	186	194	202	210	218	225	233	241	249	256	264	272	280	287	295	303	311	319	326	334	342	350	358	365	373	381	389	396	404	412	420
75	152	160	168	176	184	192	200	208	216	224	232	240	248	256	264	272	279	287	295	303	311	319	327	335	343	351	359	367	375	383	391	399	407	415	423	431
76	156	164	172	180	189	197	205	213	221	230	238	246	254	263	271	279	287	295	304	312	320	328	336	344	353	361	369	377	385	394	402	410	418	426	435	443

Source: Adapted from *Clinical Guidelines on the Identification, Evaluation, and Treatment of Overweight and Obesity in Adults: The Evidence Report.*

Acknowledgments

Writing *The Start Here Diet* has been an exciting, challenging, and awe-inspiring journey, and I would like to thank all who made this miracle happen, including first and foremost, my agent extraordinaire, Yfat Reiss Gendell of Foundry Literary + Media; my steadfast and wise editor at Ballantine, Marnie Cochran; and my collaborator and co-author, Billie Fitzpatrick, for her skill at the craft of writing and capturing the truth of who I am.

Many others at Ballantine and Random House also contributed their time and talents to this enterprise, including president and publisher of the Random House Publishing Group, Gina Centrello; Libby McGuire, publisher, Ballantine Bantam Dell; Jennie Tung, editorial director; Nina Shield, assistant editor; Crystal Velasquez, production editor; Thomas Ng, jacket designer; Virginia Norey, associate design director; and Lisa Barnes, assistant director of publicity.

A huge thank-you and appreciation go to others at the Foundry Literary + Media team, including Kirsten Neuhaus, foreign rights director; Stephanie Abou, former foreign rights director; Rachel Hecht; Sara DeNobrega; and Erica Walker.

I received wonderful support from the RKPublishing team, who understand completely the plight of all who wish to become fitter and healthier. Words do make a difference.

Thank you too, to Kierstin Buchner, whose food expertise has been invaluable.

Last but not least, I wish to thank my beloved late husband, Robert Kennedy, and my irreplaceable daughters—Rachel, Kierstin, Kelsey-Lynn, and Chelsea; this book is from them and for them.

Index

Page numbers in italic type indicate main recipe locations

About the Author

TOSCA RENO is the *New York Times* bestselling author of *Your Best Body Now* and the *Eat-Clean Diet*® series, which has sold more than two million copies worldwide. In her multiple roles as author, certified Nutritional Therapy Practitioner, fitness model, and motivational speaker, Tosca translates healthy eating into an easily adaptable and enjoyable lifestyle that has attracted big-name celebrity followers such as Angelina Jolie, Bobbi Brown, and Nicole Kidman.

She sits on the board for the Nutritional Therapy Association (NTA) and the Canadian College of Naturopathic Medicine (CCNM) and has also been a guest on numerous national TV, radio, and web programs, including *The Suzanne Show, Good Morning America, The Doctors, The Early Show* on CBS, and *Fox and Friends*.

www.toscareno.com

About the Type

This book was set in Legacy, a typeface family designed by Ronald Arnholm (b. 1939) and issued in digital form by ITC in 1992. Both its serifed and unserifed versions are based on an original type created by the French punchcutter Nicholas Jenson in the late fifteenth century. While Legacy tends to differ from Jenson's original in its proportions, it maintains much of the latter's characteristic modulations in stroke.